GOODBYE, GOOD NIGHT

KENT SMITH

ISBN: 979-8-9867100-0-6 (paperback)
Library of Congress Control Number: 2022914373

Published by KSmithBooks.com
290 E John Carpenter Frwy, #2700
Irving, TX 75062

Edited by Magnifico Manuscripts, LLC
www.magnificomanuscripts.com

Cover and InteriorDesign/Layout by MINDtheMARGINS, LLC
www.mindthemargins.com
Cover images courtesy of Freepik (rawpixel.com) and Pexels.

Printed in the United States.

To my mentors in the field of sleep medicine
who have illuminated the way:
Remmers, Rogers, Parker, Glassman, Viviano, Abramson,
Thornton, Carstensen, Spencer, Tache, Nierman
and many others.

And to those who walk the lit path with me daily:
Horn, Fields, Ring, Wilson, Schwartz, Rodgers, Mogell, Rohatgi,
Layman, Tierney, Craig, Blixt, Woltman, Liptak, Murphy, Vogel,
Sall, Soileau, Goebel, Elliott, Ben-David, Nadeau
and many others.

Finally to DT Maxx, whose medical mystery,
The Family Who Couldn't Sleep,
inspired me to create this story.

PROLOGUE

He worried about April, about the small amount in his retirement plan and about the Sea Ray Sundancer 320 Coupe he had just bought for cruising on Lake Powell. He worried about his parents' reaction.

He thought back to his fifth birthday party when, after his mother had removed his blindfold, he was surprised by a rocking horse he named King Prancer. He recalled his first girlfriend and how he tried to show off by tightroping the bicycle rack, only to slip and collapse in embarrassing agony. He remembered his years in Boy Scouts building bridges—something as an adult he had failed to do. And of course, he thought about the pain. His golden doodle, Remington, prostrated six feet away, paws under his chin, eyes canted in his direction, curious.

A drop of sweat trickled to the corner of his mouth as he said a silent prayer April would forgive him and discover another to love. *Carry on, Enzo and Luca.*

The chair fell, and the noose made of clothesline became taut. He struggled to touch the floor and futilely worked at his hands, lashed by chicken wire behind him. Other memories flew by in fuzzy detail, and after an excruciating passage of seconds, his eyes rolled back. His heart seized.

Remington whimpered, standing next to his master, nudging the legs that for years had accompanied him on daily walks to the dog park; the legs he had frequently but lazily plopped his head on as his master watched his Utah Jazz play, hoping for a loving stroke; the legs that now hung limp.

1

Memphis, Tennessee

It had been a long night. Walter's symptoms climbed to another uncomfortable level. Hallucinatory outbursts were not unusual for Sharon to see recently, but he head-butted the grandmother clock, knocking the pendulum off the hook, and asked repeatedly why the gun club was skinny-dipping in his hot tub. One minute, he made sense, but the lucidity never lasted long. He sang nursery rhymes; his favorite was, "Wheels on the Bus." And he had not slept. Not at all.

Calls to their family doctor brought prescription after prescription—Ambien, Lunesta, Trazadone, Belsomra, melatonin, NyQuil, Tylenol PM. Nothing helped. A referral to Dr. Austin, who tried cognitive behavioral therapy for insomnia, also proved fruitless.

Sharon was getting more worried as his pupils shrank to a pinpoint over the last three days. His awareness of the surroundings plummeted into a vast wasteland of shrouded memories and colorless obstacles.

A short six months ago, Walter's health was not a concern. Six feet, four inches, broad-shouldered, and two hundred twenty pounds, he had been a rugby player in college. He later taught history at Juniper High for twenty years, trying for the first fifteen to get their rugby program off the ground. He mused, "It would have been easier to burp a baby elephant." After his teaching stint, he moved in a different direction and became president of the National Council of Social Studies, where he was tasked with traveling to historical sites and educating those interested in visiting the past. Just before the sickness controlled his life, he had flown to South Fork Ranch in Parker, Texas, a few miles north of Dallas, to host an Indian wedding celebration with over four hundred attendees and a budget of two million. Toward the end of the event, he had found it difficult to walk. Many in attendance wondered what was wrong with the big-bearded host, but Sharon collected him and brought him back to the Cambria Hotel in Richardson, calling Dr. Witherspoon on the way.

"Dunhill Family Clinic. This is Rose. How can I help you?"

"This is Sharon Jenkins. Walter's wife. He's acting very odd. Might be an inner ear infection because his equilibrium is off, and he's struggling to walk."

"Can you bring him in?"

"No, we're in Dallas. Can we make an appointment tomorrow afternoon? We're flying in around noon. I can bring him straight there."

Sharon's father and brother were both physicians, and she started nursing school but made the tough decision to drop out when she realized it was not going to fulfill her like she had hoped. She and Walter had moved to Tennessee when he was offered the job at Juniper, and she found a job working the counter at a local boutique store, which allowed them to carpool on most days. She missed Laramie, Wyoming . . . missed it daily. But she loved Walter and would go anywhere with him.

"Okay, bring him in at two and we'll make it work. I have his date of birth as February 21, 1969. Is that correct?"

"Yes."

"Great. We'll see Mr. Jenkins at two tomorrow. Have a nice day!"

That was how it all started. Walter had turned fifty-two this year, and it had been the worst year of his life. Shortly after his birthday, his blood pressure and pulse became elevated in non-stressful situations, and he would start sweating without any activity. He was losing five pounds a week and developed dark circles under his eyes. His face was drawing up gradually, giving him a prunish appearance, which scared Sharon.

When she brought him in to see Dr. Witherspoon, the concerned physician concealed his disquietude. He excused himself and went to his private office to consult his resources but returned with no answers. Showing a reassuring smile, he prescribed an antidepressant and a sleep aid and told them this should pass.

Over the last week, the hallucinations had started. He walked with extreme difficulty and could not speak, other than nursery rhymes, and he developed a fever that refused to break. Dr. Witherspoon came by a few times after he got off work to check on Walter, but he was stumped.

Pulling Sharon away on his last visit, he said, "Mrs. Jenkins, this resembles an early form of dementia . . . I'm . . . not sure anything can be done. When you admitted him to the hospital a few weeks ago, they did everything they could. I don't know where this is headed, but I've made calls to some of my peers and to Vanderbilt, and oddly enough, there are a few other reports of people about Walter's age with the same progression of symptoms. All I can suggest right now is to make him as comfortable as possible."

Two days later, he was dead.

2

Baltimore, Maryland

Kendra Smeltzer had served time in the army, and when she was stationed at Fort Sill in Oklahoma, she saw a group of soldiers get struck by lightning, killing seven. One was thrown far enough to have landed at Kendra's feet, and the women who weren't killed were severely burned when the lightning traveled through the metal in their bras. This episode led her to a psychiatrist and a new diagnosis of chronic insomnia.

Two years later, her house was struck by lightning, and this threw her sleep into an unrecognizable pattern.

Soon, she developed the inability to sleep on Tuesdays and Thursdays, so when the manifestation of her insomnia took a negative turn, she did not consider it unusual.

Her husband grew so accustomed to her bouts of sleepless-ness, he considered it akin to a cosmic event when she did sleep. When she added more days than Tuesdays and Thursdays to her sleepless nights, it went unnoticed, at least until she developed new symptoms. Her face began drawing up, and the pounds were dropping off daily. She was getting clumsier, and one day she fell, fully clothed, into a full tub occupied by her husband.

"Are you drunk?" he asked, as he helped her out of the tub.

"I just lost my balance." She attempted to leave the bathroom on the water-spattered floor but fell again, this time falling face first against the toilet bowl. She collapsed and did not move, blood oozing out of her mouth.

"Kendra? Kendra!"

She would never respond nor ever know this was a kinder death than she would have experienced over the next few months.

3

Excerpt from the *Arizona Times Herald*, May 4, 2021.

Two noted authorities, on condition of anonymity, have reported no less than 18 deaths in the last week that can be traced to unexplained and extended bouts of insomnia. Experts in sleep medicine have told the Herald that sleep is vital to life and any period over seven days without sleep could lead to a medley of symptoms, including, but not limited to, severe mood swings, memory issues, trouble with thought processes, concentration, and balance, leading to accidents. Autopsies have been ordered on all who have fallen prey to this sleep thief.

Phoenix, Arizona

Kyle's trip to the office each day consisted of retracting the sunroof to accommodate his long torso, revving the speedometer to eighty-five miles an hour, edging the top of his head through the opening, connecting his phone to Apple Play, and cranking up the volume to max as he sang along with Don Henley.

He didn't care if walkers heard his serenade. He welcomed Phoenix to the Hotel California and sang of the Tiffany-twisted woman with Mercedes bends, who danced to forget. But the highway was not dark, he owned no hair for the cool wind to disturb, and he could not dance. It was his moment of departure; his statement to the world he was not the staid doctor with bursitis, grandkids, and a healthy retirement fund . . . at least for six-and-a-half minutes every weekday morning.

After his daily sojourn into rebellion, he would punch in his opera channel for the final seventeen minutes, transiently glancing in the rearview mirror to remind him who he was. The mustache was gone now, removed this morning in the aftermath of an argument with Kristy over his aversion to be transparent to the world. The "stache" he grew at age sixteen had hidden his cleft lip for the last forty-five years.

"No one will even notice," she had promised.

Tangerine trees in the median flanked him on his left while shops, restaurants, and financial institutions whisked by on his right. He pulled his midnight-blue Audi Q7 into the parking lot, where his reserved spot was very unreserved.

I can't believe she did it again, he thought.

He reluctantly found a spot with no protection from the formidable sun, unwound his six-foot, eight-inch frame from the vehicle, and took the elevator to the third floor. He officed in a five-story medical building owned by BMQ Holdings, Inc. They owned properties throughout the Phoenix area and recently had moved their headquarters from Laguna Beach for political reasons . . . at least that was the rumor. Dr. Westmoreland the dermatologist, was across the hall, Dr. Roy the dentist to his right, and Dr. Patel the obstetrician to his left. They had a good, four-year poker-playing relationship going, although recently, social media erupted over a claim Westmoreland was lecturing his dermatology patients on the evils of tattoos.

"Good morning, Dr. Hunter."

"Mornin', Nan."

"What'd you do with your lip?"

Kyle sighed. "Can you call Kristy and tell her this looks hideous?"

Nan held her chin with her left hand and squinted her emerald-green eyes. "I think it makes you look younger."

"Why do women always stick together?"

"Because—"

"Never mind. I already know the answer, and by the way, she did it again."

"You'll have to give me a little more context."

"Georgina. She parked in my spot again."

Nan rolled her eyes. "You know she's creeping up on eighty. Don't you think we should give her a break?"

Kyle shook his head as he set his Montblanc attaché beside the oak desk in his private office, then placed his fedora on the wooden hat rack in the corner. He still carried the same brief case given to him by his Aunt Merene as a high school graduation gift.

She had inherited a golf course, a diamond store, and a stable of thoroughbred horses from her late husband. Since Kyle was her favorite nephew, she had filled the case with bonds that would mature in thirty years, long after she would be gone, but soon enough for Kyle to enjoy the money. He already received a nice-enough sum from the interest every six months to allow him to live a comfortable life and to practice medicine for pleasure. When Medicare dropped the payments by fifty percent on most of the codes his office used, he just shrugged. But he did not shrug off the use of his parking spot.

"Being eighty does not absolve one from being insolent. Can you please leave a note under her windshield wiper?"

"It hasn't worked the last four times," Nan said matter-of-factly, "but I'm happy to leave another one. Should I sign it with your name this time?"

"Lord, no. She's been here sixty years and shakes hands with all the office skeletons daily. The last thing I need is for her to get sideways with me."

Nan was Kyle's physician assistant and office manager, who had been with him for over thirty years. She had joined Kyle after his dad, Dr. John Paul Hunter, retired and moved to Costa Rica to open a volunteer clinic.

"All right. I'll leave another message," Nan said with little enthusiasm. "By the way, I brought some new artwork today to *zhuzh* up the waiting room."

"Is that a new scrabble word for you?" Nan prided herself in taking on all comers in the scrabble app, *Words with Friends*.

"No comment." She dropped an air mic, swung a tight brown ponytail, and retreated to her office to pen the seventh note this month to Georgina. Nan had been the youngest cardiothoracic surgeon in her native country of El Salvador. However, civil unrest and economic instability that led to a twelve-year Salvadoran civil war became a catalyst for her immigration to the United States, her parents in tow. For a while, she considered a return to medical school, but her ailing mother's daily needs would not allow it.

Their practice weathered the corona storm and recently became busy again as patients itched to return to normalcy. They retained an older patient base because the elder Dr. Hunter had passed down his patients to Kyle, who now neared retirement age as well. Without intent, his was now a geriatric practice, and they all knew Georgina.

Over the years, they had outfitted the office with three wheelchairs and four defibrillators, but they had been profiled in several magazines for an odd collection started by the elder Dr. Hunter. No one knew what started the unusual accumulation of walking canes, but on every wall in the office hung the canes of patients who had passed on, and with the pandemic, the collection grew with a greater pace. Some were handmade and delicately carved, some topped with dragons, cobras, lions, rams, and other wild animals, a few with the Virgin Mary in place of the handle, and one with an eight ball on the end.

Kyle turned on his desktop computer and settled in to read through the charts of the day's patients. It was the usual slate of aches and pains: hypertension checks and diabetes monitoring, except for the 1:30 p.m. patient: Harold Bancroft.

Hmm. Harold never comes in. Last time I saw him in CVS, he even bragged to me about it. Insomnia. Yep, in his fifties now. Shouldn't be a problem.

When he observed Harold, he didn't like what he saw. "How we doin' today, buddy?" Harold's pupils were small, he had lost considerable weight since the CVS encounter, and there were bags under his eyes.

"I can't sleep, doc," Harold said weakly under a slumped head. This was not the energetic and grandiose Harold he had known for twenty-five years.

"That's obvious. Tell me what *you* think is going on." Kyle motioned to his medical assistant, Stephanie, to take notes.

"Don't . . . know. Haven't . . . changed anything." His speaking was labored, and he seemed to call up a reserve of energy for each word. "Diet's . . . same. Still . . . playing tennis. . . until . . . few weeks ago."

"This been going on for two weeks?" Kyle uneasily straightened his back on the four-legged stool his dad had used. The leather seat had been replaced a few times, but he could never see supplanting it.

"Hate coming . . . to the doc . . . nothing personal . . . thought it'd go away . . . Sooner or later . . . my body . . . would say, . . . 'Dude! . . . You got to sleep!' . . . And then I'd sleep . . . nope . . . Not happening. . . exhausted."

"I'm sure this is just some type of adjustment or acute insomnia," Kyle said, not sure at all. "Have you had any type of traumatic event, job change, family member dying . . . you know, that kind of stressor?"

Harold shook his head, lacking the stamina and inclination to respond.

"I'm gonna prescribe something to help you sleep." He withdrew a pen and pad from his clinic jacket and scribbled a prescription. "Don't worry. It's not anything you'll have to take forever. We just have to get you past this episode."

He nodded his head without lifting it. "Thanks, Doc. I owe ya."

4

Mobile, Alabama

Elzin Johnson loved his job on the garbage truck, and his job loved him. Mr. Peterson gave him a paper bag every Thursday morning that contained a piece of fruit, usually an apple or peach, a bottle of water, and a Danish. Rain or shine, he would shuffle out to the curb and Elzin would graciously accept it, high-fiving his eighty-five-year-old friend. Ms. Gomez gave him a candy bar every Wednesday, and the homeschooled Harkless twin boys ran out every Monday morning to give him a twin pair of twinkies. These were the regulars, but many more who loved the effervescent and engaging Elzin took much joy in feeding him, feeding him until he ballooned to three hundred and eighty pounds. Elzin didn't care. He loved his job, but not so much the dogs that growled when he would yank the garbage bags away and toss them into the RCV. They would often chase the truck as it pulled away, but he carried twinkies and apples to distract them from the smell of the refuse.

He never missed a day of work, so when he was a no-show one day, the twins asked, "Where's uncle Elzin?"

"He's just takin' a break from you guys," his partner Toby teased.

But Elzin never rode the RCV again. He went days without sleep, and at one point, fell off the truck from exhaustion and fractured his ulna. By the time it healed enough to pick up a trash bag, he was a walking zombie. His balance would remind someone of a grandma on ice skates for the first time. When he finally succumbed to what authorities were calling the insomnia flu or InF, all the weight his fans gave him had disappeared. His funeral at Belleview Baptist was standing room only, and the truck he rode for twenty-two years installed an American flag that flew at half-mast for twenty-two days.

5

Bozeman, Montana

"The dominoes are falling."

Bill Tumey, Enzo Caputo, Henry Carmichael, and Hashtag Wareness huddled around the circular table for their monthly meeting at the IHOP on 19th Street in Bozeman. It was a warmer day than usual, and on a Saturday, many students from Montana State were cycling or hiking in groups. Others hung around the parks and enjoyed the local weed they could not get in their own state or took in a show at the theaters, which had recently reopened.

The huddled group at the corner table, seated below a reprinted landscape by Ralph DeCamp, fit none of those categories. Enzo closed some blinds as the early morning eastern sun streaked their tablecloth. This drew some temporal glances from a few distracted diners, who quickly resumed their consumption of cinnamon-maple pancakes, the house specialty. Four waitresses scurried about, wiping their hands on soiled aprons after serving platters of omelets, bacon, fried eggs, hash browns, and the ubiquitous hotcakes. An elk head protruded from a wall behind the cashier, and its eyes rotated, appearing to scan the restaurant for evildoers. No one seemed to be troubled by the obtrusive or comedic intent.

Hashtag came with the news. She spoke with just enough volume to travel the few feet separating their group, her long, gray-streaked, black hair falling from her ears to cover most of her face as she leaned into their circle of trust. "I checked the database yesterday." She held up seven fingers and nodded the confirmation. There would be few words spoken this morning.

"It's really happening," Bill said.

Enzo was next. "I have the most to lose if this blows up. Be disappearing into the mountains if it does. You guys know the lodge, right?"

They all nodded and leaned back as the waiter brought their breakfast, turning the conversation to fishing.

"Hittin' the Gatlin again today, Bill?" Henry grew up in Bozeman and had been fly fishing since he was four. He went to Montana State for a degree in natural resource management, getting into politics during his sophomore year.

When the waiter left, Hashtag continued. "I think it's time to move these to weekly meetings. I know it's a longer drive for you, Enzo, but the landscape's moving rapidly, and since we can't use emails or phone calls . . ."

Hashtag moved to Montana from Searcy, Arkansas, where she was born to immigrant farmers and orphaned at six when a seventeen-year-old drunk driver killed her parents. She ricocheted between four foster families, lived in a children's home, and was sexually abused by an uncle. She ran away at sixteen, landing in Montana, where she would eventually meet the three young men, forging a meaningful relationship for the first time in her life. Born under the name Greta Pierce, she changed her name to Hashtag

Teraza Wareness after her move to the big sky. She needed to cleave her past, though her therapist discouraged it.

"Weekly meetings sound good to me, Hashy." Bill nodded in agreement. He was a poly-sci major at Rutgers. The son of a state senator, he attempted to follow in his father's footsteps, but the acrimonious dialogues and disingenuous players produced a disenfranchised student. At nineteen, he had moved to nearby Livingston to distance himself from the congested and harried northeast and open a marijuana dispensary called *The Joint Joint*.

"I'll do my best," said Enzo. "Sachi knows nothing and might ask questions, but I think she'll be fine." Enzo traveled the farthest to live in the area. Born to a mother who was a hospitalist physician and a father who was a genomics researcher, he was expected to pursue a field in the sciences, and he did not disappoint. Growing up with his father's research, he became fascinated with the industry-wide focus on developing new cures for pesky and forgotten diseases. He came to the states from the Veneto region of Italy at twenty-four and landed at Rutgers, where he established a friendship with Bill. The only one to have married so far among their quartet, he persuaded his bride to move to Big Sky after agreeing to move her mother, too.

"You all have the log in to the Google drive?" Hashy asked. They each nodded.

"Great. Check it daily." The conversation edged close to silence as they ate, and scarcely heightened as they readied to tab out.

"See everyone next Tuesday? Same time?" Bill asked. They each gave a thumbs-up and hurried to their cars, not because there was a sudden and unexpected chill in the air signaling an unusual cool front, but because they felt a quick exit would allow their hushed conversation to dissolve into the leftover pancakes.

6

Phoenix, Arizona

"Hey, boss, can I come in?"

Jacob Potter's door was slightly ajar, and Bowlsby wanted to know about the company party on Friday. Although Jacob's family owned the *Arizona Times Herald*, he was a hands-on owner and took on the role of managing editor five years ago. Critics in the profession publicly questioned the decision in 2016, but over time the castigations softened until they were replaced by adulations. The Century Building, home to the *Arizona Times Herald* since it was erected in 1921, was remodeled in 1946, then again in 1953 after lightning struck an antenna on the roof and fried the wiring throughout the building. One could still smell bouquets of cigar smoke in the walls from the chain-smoking reporters in the last half-century.

"Please, Tom." Jacob motioned, not glancing up from the manuscript he was reading.

"Sorry to bother you, but what's the policy this year on dates to the party?"

Morale at the *Arizona Times Herald* had been on the rise lately with their only formidable competition filing Chapter 11, and advertisers leaving for more fertile ground. They, too, were dangerously close to shutting down, furloughing three journalists, two copywriters, and even Shakespeare, a janitor who was an institution at the *Arizona Times Herald* for thirty-seven years.

On his eighteenth birthday, Keith Rockett was inspired to memorize *Macbeth* and inserted phrases from the play in scores of situations over the years, earning the name Shakespeare for good reason. When Danny King, five feet, four inches with platform shoes, was promoted to executive editor in 2008, Shakespeare stood on a stepstool, out of Danny's earshot, and quoted in his best Shakespearean brogue.

"Now does he feel his title hang loose about him, like a giant's robe upon a dwarfish thief." His job security teetered after that, but he hung on until the recent cut.

Jacob Potter decided this was the right time to announce a celebration party at his uncle's estate. Sidney Potter once owned the *Arizona Times Herald* in better days before the internet supplanted the reading eyes of the younger public, and the older public was shrinking quicker than the Phoenix paper wanted to admit. It was Jacob's grandfather, Bunyan, who built the *Arizona Times Herald,* and they kept it in the family. Jacob was well respected by the staff, primarily due to his approachability, and less so for his propriety.

"Yes, of course, Tom. Don't suppose you'll be bringing the redhead?" He grinned, showing the reassuring smile they all loved. "Looking forward to meeting her."

"Thanks, and yes, I'll be bringing Marta. By the way, I know Sylvia wouldn't want me to say anything, but she looked awful today."

Sylvia Witherspoon, the managing editor for the last twenty-two years, had won four Bradlees, more than any other editor in the fifty states. Her work on the Enron bankruptcy and the Boston marathon bombing won critical acclaim. A few days ago, she had brought her three-year-old granddaughter for Bring Your Daughter to Work Day, and the staff fawned over the youngster until she pulled over the popcorn machine, scattering broken glass and buttered Orville Redenbacher over the break-room floor. The embarrassment and the shard of glass embedded in little Heather's hand sent both home. Sylvia had not been the same editor since.

"What do you mean?" Jacob asked.

Tom Bowlsby walked farther into the room and closed the door. "She's saying things that don't make sense."

"Like what?" Jacob dropped the manuscript on the desk, walked around, and sat on the edge, arms folded across his chest, his taut and tanned face showing genuine concern.

"Larry asked her about the deadline on the chemical ware-house explosion, and she mumbled something no one could understand. We all tried not to listen, but the awkwardness was palpable. It was like a train wreck."

"That doesn't sound too bad," Jacob said, hoping for a better explanation.

"She was acting drunk."

"She doesn't drink."

"That's my point. She was sweating through her blouse. She called Mike, Phillip, and she's known Mike for over five years. There's trash all around her wastebasket. It's like she kept missing it on purpose."

"Did someone urge her to go home?" Jacob opened the blinds covering the glass in his office and surveyed the milieu on the floor.

"We didn't have to. She realized she wasn't herself and left, but it was scary seeing her get into the elevator."

"You let her leave by herself?" Jacob ran out the door toward the elevator, Tom following close behind. As they reached the unparted door and waited, Jacob turned to Tom. "You mean no one went with her? Offered to drive her home?"

Tom meekly shook his head. He had been hired as Jacob Potter's assistant after the third female in a row became pregnant and decided to stay home with their newborn. There were twelve applicants: eleven females and Tom. He graduated from the Medill School of Journalism at Northwestern and, rather than apply for the graduate program, he headed to Phoenix to follow the redhead and applied with the *Arizona Times Herald*. The interview was short, and he started the next day.

The elevator arrived and dropped them seven floors. When the doors opened, they witnessed the flashing lights of a police car through the glass doors in the front of the building. They raced outside just in time to see Sylvia's blank eyes staring out the rear window as the police car drove away into an afternoon sprinkle.

"You know that lady?" asked a gawking, pimple-faced teenage boy holding a skateboard under his right arm.

"Yes, why?" asked Jacob, visibly shaken.

"Cops thought she was baked."

"Excuse me?"

"On marijuana," said Tom.

"Oh."

Pimples said, "Yeh. She was stumbling around, saying some incoherent shit. She didn't put up much of a fight. Just let the cops cuff her and put her into the car. You guys got any of what she was on?" he asked.

"Scram, kid," Jacob said, showing restraint. He wanted to smack the acne off the teen's face. "Tom, find out where they're taking her. I've got some calls to make." He whirled and bolted back through the glass doors.

Growing up, Jacob's family lived in the city, but Uncle Sidney lived on a sprawling, four-hundred-acre ranch outside of Phoenix, which juxtaposed with the reservation of the Salt River Pima-Maricopa Indian Community. He would spend a few weeks each summer learning how to take care of livestock, bail hay, and kill rattlesnakes with his .22.

Some days, he longed to be twelve again, free from the encumbrances of being in charge.

7

Dallas, Texas

Carol Bleeker was a kept woman, or at least that was how she introduced herself at parties. Her husband was a successful stockbroker, and they lived on Lake Cypress where the most affordable homes brought eight figures, all before the decimal. She taught third grade in Belton, Texas, early on, but Oliver, twelve years her senior, spirited her away to Dallas.

Today, Oliver came home early from the office, which rarely happened unless he was changing clothes to play golf with his college roommates from Rice University. Not today. He had not been Oliver lately. He'd been distant, sometimes confused, and staying up much later than he had done in many years.

"Honey, what's going on?"

"I don't know. It's like someone injected me with a rogue bottle of caffeine. I can't get any sleep lately, and it's affecting my work."

"Have you contacted Dr. Jenkins?"

He loosened his BVLGARI silk tie as she motioned him to sit on the couch in their spacious parlor.

"Bethany called for me. Got me an appointment on Wednesday, but the nurse told her I was the third patient with these symptoms this week."

"I guess the Ambien he gave you last year when your mother passed are gone?"

"I never took them back then. I wasn't that upset," he said, with as much sarcasm as he could muster. "I did take one a few nights ago, and it didn't help. Took two last night and never slept. This can't go on."

That evening, Carol searched online to see what could be creating his symptoms, and it was scary. Nothing came up in PubMed or WebMD. Mainstream media had to be conservative in their reporting.

Dallas News, June 3, 2021.

Just after wrestling COVID-19 into submission, authorities are now working with epidemiologists to discover what is bringing these cases of insomnia to our middle-aged citizens. Is it genetic? Is it transmitted through respiratory channels? Something in the water? Diet? There is much speculation, and the CDC as well as the NIAID are working around the clock to get a handle on this new challenge we now face. At present, it is prudent to self-isolate when you can, particularly those persons in their 50s, until we can get a better handle on both causation and a potential cure.

Alternate sources were more incendiary. One tub-thumper summarized:

The Peabody Press, June 3, 2021.

Fact: Twenty-three million will die. If you are in your 50s, there is little doubt you will contract the new insomnia disease InF. There are 23 million Americans in this age group, and we add 63,000 to that age group every day. If you are in this demographic, insurance agents are not answering your emails and are inventing loopholes to cancel your policy. Act now. Visit www.NoSleepLawyers.com for a free consultation. We will fight for YOU!

They had been sleeping separately for the last seven years. His snoring drove her to the guest room, but even after he got this controlled with a device from a sleep dentist, they slept apart. He liked sleeping with their retriever. She did not. He liked the thermostat at sixty-five. She liked seventy-two. He needed a pitch-black bedroom. She liked a night light. But she always knew when he went to bed . . . or when he did not. The next morning, she realized he had not.

She found him sitting in a lounge chair by the pool. As she approached him, he turned and said, "Jack's coming by at ten. Didn't want to surprise you."

"Didn't know attorneys worked on Saturdays."

"He owes me. I got him tickets to the Masters, and the sumbitch never paid me for 'em."

"I don't remember you going to the Masters. I thought it was the U.S. Open."

Oliver hung his head and slowly swung it side to side. "Just need sleep."

"Think we can move that appointment up from Wednesday? Was that the soonest Jenkins's office could get you in?"

He made no effort to raise his head, and he was not responding.

"Oliver? Honey?"

"I'm trying to remember. I really am. I'm sure I have meetings on Monday and Tuesday, but I can't remember anything about them."

"Oliver!" Jack rounded the corner of the house and approached the couple.

"Carol, can you give us some privacy? It's a confidential matter." This was a usual occurrence with her husband. He was on countless boards and ran three companies, so she was already standing and nodding to the attorney.

"Good to see you, Jack. Would you like anything to drink?"

"I'm good, Carol. Shouldn't be long." He sat in the chair she had just vacated, looking uncomfortable in a suit and tie.

"All right. I'll be inside if you change your mind." When she disappeared into the house, Oliver turned to Jack.

"I told you this was about shoring up my will, but I have a serious question."

"Should I ask Carol for that drink? Maybe a scotch? A double?"

"I just need to know one thing, and I'm calling attorney-client privilege."

"Jesus, Oliver."

"I'm serious. This goes no further."

"All right. I promise." Jack loosened his tie, sensing this could take some time.

"Does anything change in the will if my death is ruled a suicide?"

"Oh, Christ. Please—"

"When did you get religion, Jack?"

"What does that—"

"Never mind. Just answer my question and dispense with the histrionics."

"Only your life insurance, but with your net worth, I doubt that's a concern. Will you let me call my sister?"

"Don't need a shrink, counselor. It was only a theoretical question. Nothing but."

Carol poked her head out the partially opened back door. "Changed your mind, Jack?" She was used to seeing the attorney with a drink in hand, provided it was after noon. It was only 10:00 a.m., but she recognized the angst on his face.

"Double scotch, on the rocks! No, make it neat."

After Oliver's tenth consecutive night of no sleep, he walked into his bathroom, locked the door, picked up his razor, laid down in the porcelain bathtub, and slit both wrists.

That night, he slept.

8

Phoenix, Arizona

Another one? Kyle stared into his laptop, scrolling across his schedule for the day.

> 9:15 - Fred Winters, insomnia, fever.
> 11:50 - Suzanne Hampton, insomnia, equilibrium/dizziness.

What's going on? That's three in two days. He opened all three charts to probe for similarities. *Two males and one female . . . one on a beta blocker . . . one obese . . . one on Viagra . . . one on hormone therapy . . . They're all about the same age—fifty-one, fifty-four, and fifty-six. Age is the only variable they have in common.*

Kyle shunned anecdotal evidence, and an *n* of three did not constitute research, but it was all he had to go on. A graduate of Dartmouth, he had been accepted at the school of medicine at Johns Hopkins, but when his mother died from breast cancer, which metastasized to most of her lymph nodes, he decided on the University of Arizona College of Medicine at Phoenix so he could be close to his father.

The elder Dr. Hunter was a pioneer in the embryonic research into smoking as a causative factor in cancer and was in some combustible wars against the powerful tobacco lobbies. He sported "more bruises than a frog has warts," he was fond of claiming, but it never deterred him. Almost thirty years later, Kyle had battled the errant, fear-based claims surrounding AIDS. He picked up his phone and punched line thirty-two.

"What do you need, Dr. Hunter?"

"Nan, could you pull the bloodwork on Fred Winters, Suzanne Hampton, and Harold Bancroft?"

"On it."

"Aren't you going to ask why?" Kyle asked.

"Not really. I'm sure you have your reasons. I'll have them on your desk in ten minutes."

Kyle wondered how he would survive without Nan. She hinted at retirement recently, but he rebuffed the overtures and said she could retire when he did. In seven minutes, she knocked on his door and entered without a response from the lanky doctor.

"Here you are. May I *now* ask why you needed these three?" She gave him a mischievous smile.

He acknowledged her and grinned. "Nope." After she left, he went through their lab work in detail. *Nothing unusual. Hampton's hematocrit is up, but she's overweight . . . likely sleep apnea . . . makes sense. Thyroid levels all good. Hampton a little low in Vitamin D . . .* Dead end.

9

The *Arizona Times Herald* office party was held at the JW Marriott Phoenix Desert Ridge Resort and Spa, and Jacob released his HR manager, Cameron for the day to get everything set up. He vacillated on how to approach the festivities with Sylvia's unusual condition weighing on the team, but decided his people needed a distraction and a celebration for weathering the economic hiccough. His only instructions to Cameron were to have the hotel set the thermostat to sixty-seven degrees and to remove any clocks.

"Thanks for coming!" Jacob reached out to shake hands with Kyle. "And who is this pretty lady on your arm?" He grinned as he leaned and kissed Kristy on a perfumed cheek.

"My better half," Kyle said. "Sorry we're early, but Kristy's had a long day, so I promised we would offer our congratulations and make it an early night."

"At least it's after five," she said, holding a half-empty glass of chardonnay up for inspection.

Kristy's work with the Red Cross spanned close to thirty years. The pandemic had taxed their resources, but a week of COVID paled in comparison to 9/11. With a disaster of that magnitude, protocol moved the call center far away from the epicenter. She was transferred to Dallas, tasked with coordinating all calls coming in, and triaging them in a timely manner. She slept very little during the week following the tragedy, but those days forged in her the belief if she could survive that week, she could breeze through every other challenge. Today, she handled calls from the House Energy and Commerce Oversight Panel regarding recently uncovered mismanaged funds. She escaped with a battered but intact dignity. The Red Cross was singled out for opprobrium in the aftermath of 9/11, so she knew when to speak and when to punt to the lawyers.

"Sleeping well, Kristy?" Jacob's wife walked up with her own glass of wine.

"Yes, why do you ask?"

"You look like you haven't slept in days."

"It's been a rough day, but I'm fine. Nothing a glass or three of wine won't take care of. Hey, this place looks fabulous. You guys know how to throw a party."

"That would be Cameron," Jacob said. "She can work some magic."

"Tell her she can decorate my place anytime."

Others began showing up, walking through a mouth-shaped hole in a thirty-foot papier-mâché blue mask. Most made their way over to ensure Jacob saw them, then angled toward the hors d'oeuvres and open bar. Tom Bowlsby, wearing a light-blue '80s-inspired tux introduced the redhead to *Arizona Times Herald* employees, then brought her to meet Jacob.

"Tom has spoken highly of you, Marta. Thanks for coming."

"The pleasure is mine. He can't say enough good things about you, Mr. Potter. You have this guy for life." She winked at Tom.

"I hope so," Jacob said.

"Who is that with Danny?" Tom motioned toward the editor and a woman wearing a shimmery, gold dress, which hugged bony outcroppings and terminated a few inches shy of modesty. Standing eight inches taller than Danny, she pointed to an item on the shelf behind the bartender.

"Where's Sheryl?"

"None of our business, Tom. I'm assuming they're separated." As if on cue, the pair approached them. The group turned toward them awkwardly, smiling with feigned authenticity.

"Hey guys!" Danny began. "This is Heidi." As she raised her dirty martini in a nice-to-meet-you gesture, the others nodded in her direction. The pouty lips framed by a porcelain face never moved. Jacob wondered if they were stuck.

"Heidi's a pharmaceutical rep for Glaxo. I plan on raiding her car trunk if you get my drift." He smiled, but in an interruption of her immobile face, she rolled her eyes. "But seriously, she knows—"

"Governor Adair! Great to see you," Jacob said as he interrupted Danny's explanation. The governor smiled and held out a hand to Jacob as he eyed Danny's date.

"Wouldn't miss it, Jacob! Your editorials haven't always been kind to me, but that's part of the job. I don't let acrimony in the press affect relationships."

Jacob smiled, knowing neither he nor Governor Adair believed that statement. Wendy was not smiling. Her opinion of the governor fluctuated between disgust and disdain. She came from a family of cannabis pioneers, her parents running three marijuana companies listed on the NYSE and NASDAQ. The governor had opposed every piece of marijuana legislation since he took office. The topic was a hot-button issue in Jacob and

Wendy's relationship as well, so they chose to embrace a tacit understanding of each other's position. The disparity began with their efforts to solve infertility twenty-five years ago. After three failed IVF attempts at ten thousand dollars each, Jacob blamed the misfortune on Wendy's use of marijuana. Wendy blamed it on his lack of marijuana use. Stalemate.

"I can't stay long," said the governor. "This f-ing Delta variant is kicking my butt."

"You've got the Delta?" asked the anorexic Heidi, backing up as she spoke.

"No, no, it's creating miles of paperwork I have to sift through. People expect me to make some decisions or at least have an opinion. Right now, all I know is people are dying. I'm just glad to see most people here are wearing masks."

"No worries," said Jacob. "I appreciate you took time out to come."

Wendy was seething as she stood by Jacob. Adair reminded her of Oswald Cobblepot on *Batman*, but she held that opinion to herself. . . usually.

Adair's phone vibrated in his pocket. He held it to his ear, then turned to Jacob. "Sorry. Have to take this. Great party!" He attached the phone to his ear again and proceeded through the glass doors to the back patio.

Wendy could no longer refrain. "Who thinks he looks like the penguin on *Batman*?"

This brought muffled laughter and Danny said, "Yes, we get letters to the editor many times that use Oswald when they're talking about the governor. It took us a minute to realize who they were referring to."

Kristy took a sip of her drink and nodded, watching the back doors. "That conversation sure looks animated."

Each of them turned to see the commotion. Governor Adair appeared to be in a heated discussion with someone on the other end. When Ted from the *Arizona Times Herald* mailroom walked through the doors to smoke a cigarette outside, Adair quickly ended the call and came back through the doors, perspiration dripping from his bushy sideburns. As the irascible man of short stature neared their group, red-faced, he bristled, "Should have run for governor in Minnesota. It's too f-ing hot in this town." He strode out the entrance without another word.

10

"I assure you. Senator Bonner is doing fine. Just a little fatigued from being on the road so much, and her doctor instructed her to take it easy, so she's not doing any pressers right now. She's also getting ready for the judiciary hearing tomorrow, but I'm happy to field any questions unrelated to her health, as I am no physician."

The press room today was SRO with more standing than sitting. Bonner's communications director, Jilian Quito, stood behind and was dwarfed by a large oak podium, which proudly displayed the great seal of the state of Arizona. She was flanked by flags of the United States on her right and of Arizona on her left.

Senator Stella Bonner was the third daughter of Cuban immigrants, who escaped to the States in July 1962 when her father, who was a military scientist, shunned Castro's communism. After the botched Bay of Pigs in 1961, he became more restless, and when he was asked to join the design team for missile launch facilities in early 1962, he planned their exodus. They lived in Miami for eighteen months, and after Stella was born, they moved to San Diego, deciding the temperate climate of Cuba was the only thing they missed.

Stella Garcia enrolled in San Diego State after high school graduation, then married Laird Bonner in the summer after her sophomore year. They were both political science majors and, after graduation, moved to Phoenix where his father was a state senator. They quickly became a power couple, and after learning they could not have children, opted to devote their careers completely to politics instead of adopting.

On a salmon fishing trip Laird took with three friends from high school, the four-seat Cessna Skyhawk he was piloting crested the top of a peak in the Cascade Mountain Range, only to discover, too late, another peak hiding under a cloud drape. There were no survivors, and by the time the plane was found, it was six days later, and the autopsy results were controversially sealed, claiming there was too little left to identify cause of death after mountain lions had done what wild carnivores do. Laird's father exerted considerable pressure to prevent any leakage. Stella's career was temporarily sidelined after this, but it did not take long for the public to embrace her, encouraging her to become the second senator named Bonner in Arizona. In the last election, she won her third term with over ninety percent of the vote.

Several questions overlayed each other, but a bass voice from the right side three rows back asked, "Does Senator Bonner have the insomnia flu?"

News was spreading about adults in their fifties contracting a disease that carried flu-like symptoms but with accompanying insomnia, which worsened each successive night. Dr. Axel Throckmorton, an epidemiologist in Pittsburgh, named it the insomnia flu or InF. He called for quarantining anyone with complaints of insomnia until they could be sure what vehicle was being used for transmission. Those earning solitary confinement were patients who displayed a combination of chronic insomnia with either delirium, equilibrium deficits, aphasia, dystonia, or a fever of 103 or higher. Quarantining received little traction, but it was gaining ground as more cases were reported.

"Next question, please!" replied Jilian.

A sonorous voice rang out from the nine o'clock position. "Has she been tested for the new flu?"

Jilian Quito lowered and slowly shook her head from side to side, then spoke into the microphone. "If there are no more questions, this press conference has concluded." She stepped down from the podium and exited among an excitable press, which continued to bellow questions.

Brent met her backstage. Thin drapes through which shadows could be seen did not prevent him from questioning her. "Ms. Quito, when is the senator gonna allow you to tell 'em?"

The spindly, freckled, young man was interning during the summer and enjoyed being edgy as he stretched the boundaries demanded of other interns. He prided himself, through a prism of naivete, in his quest to improve translucency. Jilian knew the type. They always took a few months, and more than a few dressings down by their superiors, to abandon their cause and submit to loyalty.

"In due time," the sanguine Jilian said. "In due time."

11

"What do you mean, we can't see her?" Jacob was careful to hide his press credentials, but the nurse did not budge. After he left the *Arizona Times Herald* party, he dropped Wendy off at their home and picked up a thankful Tom to go see Sylvia. After the redhead consumed her second vodka, she began flirting with Ted from the mailroom and one of the reporters named Sawyer. Tom needed an excuse to take her home, and Jacob came through.

"I'm sorry, sir, but only her family is allowed in her room," the nurse said dismissively.

"But we *are* family," Jacob said.

"Your ID?" She held out her hand.

"We're her work family," Tom said, but the nurse ignored him.

"I'm sorry, gentlemen, but rules are rules." Her head never lifted as she rifled through some sheets on her clipboard. Jacob edged closer like a shark smelling bloodied snapper.

"Nurse . . . Simmons. There's a man in 403 who's peed his sheets and no one's bothered to check on him since we arrived. From the sweet smell, he must have diabetes. Your nurse over there is eating Cheez-Its and texting. The fire extinguisher on the wall we walked by hasn't been inspected in three years, and I smelled marijuana on the elevator. I manage the *Arizona Times Herald,* and I would love to run an investigative report on the state of your hospital. Tom, did you get her name down? It's Simmons. Celia Simmons, Chief Nursing Officer, Margo Community Hospital." He glared at the stunned nurse. "Now, Ms. Simmons, do we look like family, or are you still playing hard-ass gatekeeper?"

Without saying a word, she waved them toward room 417.

Jacob had correctly assessed the condition of the hospital when he handled Nurse Simmons. The linoleum floor begged to be replaced, room numbers were missing, and sound barriers were needed. The air conditioning ductwork rattled above the ceiling tiles as the HVAC strained, unsuccessfully, to obey the commands of the control system. He noted several HIPAA violations and made a mental note that if he did an exposé, he would have more than enough material.

As he walked down the hall, his "gait song" clicked on. It started as a teenager when "Whoot, There It Is" by Quad City Knock was playing in the gym during basketball practice. When he had walked off the court, his steps were in sync with the beat of the song, and he decided he would begin doing this with every walk, whether music was playing or not. He determined what emotion he was feeling or perhaps wanted to feel, then played a song in his head to fit the situation. On this walk, his gait song was, "This is How We Do It," by Montell Jordan.

"Sylvia, what's going on?" Jacob asked, as they entered her room. A blanket of antisepsis wafted over them. He stepped around a stand holding bags dripping clear liquids into her veins. Through the token window, the setting sun casted a column of light across her torso.

"I wish I knew, but what I've heard since I was admitted is that they're two others in this hospital with my symptoms. Is this an investigative visit, or are you here to cheer me up?"

"That's the Sylvia I know," Jacob said as he sat on the edge of the hospital bed.

She had been the associate editor when Jacob took over for his uncle in 1995. He was warned she was a tiger, and early on when he approached her to follow a story where France exploded a nuclear device in the Pacific, she showed him what a real explosion looked like. Since that exchange, they became one of the most productive teams in journalism. Volatile, but the edginess kept them sharp.

"The cops thought I was on drugs. Believe me, I *wish* I were on drugs. This ain't fun."

"How long has this been going on?" He squeezed her arm gently.

"Hard to say. It's been gradual. Sleeping problems for months, but it's getting harder to focus. I'm sleeping maybe two hours a night. They have me pumped up with Modafinil right now. They said it helped others in this condition with their executive and cognitive functions, but I still can't sleep. Believe me, I feel much better now compared to when I arrived here. I did ask if we could talk to the other two in the hospital, but my request was denied."

"You should see Jacob at work in this hospital," said Tom. "I bet *he* can get interviews."

Jacob tried to conceal his concern. "You take it easy, Syl. Take all the time you need. Danny can hold down the fort, and Larry can fill in the gaps. We'll let you rest now, and I'll check back tomorrow."

"Thanks. I guess this is that insomnia flu that's been reported in some hospitals. I've been wishing that diagnosis away for a few weeks, but dammit, my genie must be on vacation."

Jacob smiled. "If anyone can beat this, you can. I'll tell the nurse to let you sleep for a few hours." He bit his lip, immediately regretting what he said.

"Uh, if you have some secret potion to get me those hours, I'll be back in the office tomorrow!"

Jacob hoped he read humor in her response, but her face revealed something quite different. Her eyes showed concern, and her chin showed fear. "I'm sure you'll be back sooner than later. Maybe you can sneak down and interview the other victims here for a start."

"On it!" she said, raising her right thumb in acknowledgment.

As he left her room, Jacob felt in some odd way that he had let her down. His self-flagellation was unearned, but she was his charge, and erringly, he felt culpable. It was a lesson he learned at a young age from his uncle Sidney, when his father's brother saved him from an angry drift of feral hogs.

Tom followed Jacob to the elevator. When the door closed, Jacob said, "I don't think she's going to be with us tomorrow."

"What are you talking about?" Tom's eyes widened as he peered up at Jacob.

"Landon's been working on a piece. He hasn't shown it to Sylvia yet. This is happening all over the US, and it's not pretty." Jacob had received hundreds of memos in the previous twelve hours from sources so varied and unexpected, he found it difficult to separate fact from absurdity. "So far, everyone exhibiting these symptoms has died or slowly deteriorates. Everyone is in Sylvia's age group and the experts are . . . well, they're confused. Now that she's become one of—"

The elevator door opened to a lobby with two inches of water covering the floor. Hospital personnel scrambled to find the cause and to stem the steady flow from the ceiling. *Unbelievable*, thought Jacob as he and Tom carefully negotiated the path to the front door.

Once they were back in Jacob's Escalade and on the road, Tom said, "You were saying? Something about Sylvia's condition?"

"Oh, yes. Now that she is likely one of the victims—"

"I wish you wouldn't word it that way."

"Sorry. There's not a better word right now. We still must run with it. We don't have a choice. If we don't, we'll be accused of sitting on a story."

This happened to Jacob's uncle Sidney in the '60s, shortly after he took over from *his* father, Bunyan. When John Lennon said the public was more infatuated with the Beatles than Jesus, he sat on the story, not knowing what perspective to take in the Bible-Belt South. Other papers ran with it, and the *Arizona Times Herald* board formally reprimanded the CEO. Jacob would not let that happen as long as he was in charge.

"The FBI sent a secure memo to eight hundred papers with the largest readership, strongly discouraging any publication relating to the insomnia flu until more was known. They're afraid of mass panic, but the subject is trending on Twitter and every other social media platform. You've likely seen rumors online in the last twelve hours."

"Yes, I have." Tom rubbed his eyes and recalled his hours of surfing until after midnight. "Some are saying this is foreign interference. Some say it's political. No one knows what to believe."

"It's the type of hysteria we see when we don't have answers, just questions, so the piece we're running is about those questions. I've already told Landon, and he's got it ready to run in the morning."

12

"Nan, can you get Dr. Jimmerson on the phone?" Kyle was getting concerned with what he was seeing in his patient base, and he knew if anyone could enlighten him, it would be his sleep-doctor friend.

After a minute, Nan buzzed Kyle. "She's on two, sir."

"Hello, Marie?"

"Hi, Kyle. How can I help you?"

"I've got three patients who—"

"Way ahead of you. Assume this is about some insomnia?"

"Yes."

"I've been seeing cases for two weeks. I have an idea what this might be but don't have the resources to run the tests. Besides, the tests aren't yet validated. Too many false positives."

"What do you think it is?"

"You familiar with prion diseases?"

"Like Mad Cow?"

"Yes, and like chronic wasting disease in deer and elk. Like Creutzfeldt-Jakob disease and like kuru in Papua New Guinea in the 1950s. The formal name for prion diseases is transmissible spongiform encephalopathies or TSEs."

"Wow. Is this what we're seeing?" He reclined his chair and threw both legs onto his desk. He could see this conversation extending long enough to give his aging back some respite.

"Too early to tell. The only definitive test is postmortem. Have you heard of CTE?"

"You mean the brain injuries football players get from being hit in the head all the time?"

"Yes. Same thing. You can only diagnose it posthumously. You can biopsy a patient's brain who you think may have a prion disease, but it's dangerous for the patient, and it could create exposure. Dissecting brain tissues on the deceased is the only acceptable method, so until we see results from autopsies, which shouldn't be too far off, the misfolded proteins—those are the hallmark of the TSEs—can't be seen."

"But which TSE are we seeing?"

"Have you heard of FFI or fatal familial insomnia?"

"No. Tell me more."

Dr. Marie Jimmerson had moved into the Phoenix area after some work at the University of Florida, where she researched testing for TSEs before the patient died. Politics and a lack of NIH funding they expected put a clamp on her studies, although she was close to some answers. With objections from her superiors and her boyfriend moving to Arizona, she headed west. She moved into the same complex as Kyle and his wife, and they had struck up a friendship when they met at the Phoenix Metro Bicycle Club. Both were avid riders.

"It's only been traced back to the 1760s in Italy because many records were lost during the Napoleonic wars. It's thought to have started with a doctor who contracted it in some unknown way, but then passed down through his lineage. That's the genetic form, but that's not how we get Mad Cow disease from cows."

"It's been a while, but from what I recall, we humans were only at risk if we consumed cows that were infected."

"Exactly. None of us are descended from cows, so there are multiple routes for transmission of prion diseases."

Kyle sucked his cheeks and squinted, something he did when concentrating. "So . . . you're saying we wouldn't know how all these people are getting it if it's this fatal familial insomnia brand of prions, right?"

"Not yet, but the people coming down with this are in their fifties primarily. That mirrors FFI and not any of the other TSEs, and as far as we know, the only way FFI can be transmitted is genetically."

"As far as we know *now*, I suppose. All these people can't be related, right?"

"Exactly. Just in my patient base, there's no relation between most. I've already seen two deaths. It's brutal." Marie shook her head. "I would never want to die like this."

"Need any patients for your database?"

"I think I'll have more than enough. Primary care docs are sending me these patients; some are finding me on their own. I don't even take lunches anymore. Appreciate this break, though, so I can talk to someone who's had some sleep lately. You're sleeping well, aren't you?"

"Yep. I'm sixty-one, so hoping I'm not in the demographic to catch this."

"We don't know yet that it's confined to the specific fifties' age group," she said carefully.

"Ouch. Okay, but I appreciate the transparency. Does anyone else know about this FFI?"

"Yes, but I don't know if they've connected the dots. To be honest, there may be no dots to connect, but I'm determined to explore the possibility. Can you keep this on the QT for now?"

"Of course, but I can't allow my patients to experience something that could have a cure, so you'll have to keep me updated. Fair?"

"Of course!"

13

"Senator, I think you need to let me say something. We can't keep putting them off." Jilian was more concerned about her friend than being transparent, but pressure was building. Her job was to protect her boss's reputation and to show a courageous face—and sometimes a façade—to the public. They were seated in the senator's ample study, which had hosted heads of state, foreign dignitaries, and of course, her nieces and nephews who she loved to spoil. She sat, wearily, at her marble-topped desk under a photo of her late husband. Jilian stood in front of her, holding an iPad with Jilian's schedule on it. There were no windows in her office. In this era of unfettered lunacy, security won out over the pleasantries and distractions of a scenic view.

"If I'm reading the tea leaves right," said Senator Bonner, "I don't have much time to make an acceptable public statement myself. I'm already struggling to control my pulse, and this is the third outfit I've had on this morning. Just can't control the sweating."

"Why don't you let me do this. I can take the heat. That's why I make the big bucks," she said, smiling weakly.

Senator Bonner was in no condition to stand in front of the media. She stumbled over words and in her last press conference, she could not remember the name of her main nemesis, Newton Ball with the *Des Moines Daily*. All she could think of was *fig*, and she came close to using it.

"You're quite persuasive, Jilian. Go ahead and okay the purse . . ."

"Press conference?"

Bonner leaned into her open hands and began to weep softly, her stringy, sweat-soaked hair sticking to her shivering wrists. "I'm not ready for this. I'm not strong enough . . . just not ready."

Jilian leaned over and hugged her, feeling bones that had once been covered with toned muscle. "I'm here for you."

She wiped her eyes, then focused on Jilian. "This shouldn't be about me. It's too late. It should be about our constitutions. . . the people, dammit."

"I'll make sure to steer it that way, Senator. Gonna watch on the monitor?"

"I don't know. I'll try."

"Either way, I'll fill you in." She kissed Jilian on a salty cheek and left the office, then leaned into her lapel mic. "Tell them it's on, but it'll be me. Just don't tell *them* that."

Before she entered the door to approach the podium, she took a deep breath. As she stepped to the mic, the barrage began.

"When is the senator making a statement?"

"What is she doing to calm the fears of the citizens?"

"Is she still alive?"

Ignoring the blather, Jilian began speaking, eyes lacking any hint of concern. She raised her hand, palm forward, hoping to quell the uprising. All it managed to do was encourage a room full of raised hands.

"Members of the press. First, I have just spoken with Senator Bonner, and I could not and would not have done so if she were dead. She is in good spirits, but she gave me one directive and one directive only. This fight is not about her. It's about every single person she represents, and on a broader scale, it's about anyone in the sightline of this awful flu. Whether she lives or dies, every waking moment for now is concentrated on being an agent for knowledge. How is this insomnia flu transmitted? Who is susceptible? Is there a cure? A vaccine? Not for her, but for you. She is on the phone twenty-three hours a day calling those in the CDC and NIAID who—"

"Twenty-three hours a day? That's some fake news!" A sarcastic voice sounded from the second row.

"If you had done your research on InF, you would know that sleep is a luxury these victims are not afforded, Mr. Bayne. As I was saying, she is in a unique position. She is experiencing first-hand what InF can do to someone, but additionally, her access to open channels is a privilege few carry. She does not take her position lightly. She is using her perspective to help those in the epidemiological trenches as they probe for answers. You want answers? So does she. So do we all, and as soon as she collects any answers, you will also have them. Thank you for your time."

She exited to a chorus of questions and a few claps of appreciation. She was thankful she had planted some of the senator's people in the press room.

14

Clyde Turrentine was struggling. His small business—a euphemism for a company with one employee—was called The Yard Barber and his slogan was, "Just a Little Off the Top." He had taken care of lawns for the last thirty years, but this summer was rough. He did not feel like himself, and his girlfriend Becky was concerned.

"Clyde, you can't keep doing this. You're not twenty-five anymore, and it's gettin' to ya. You're a ball-o-sweat when you come in, and the wreck you had today . . . it's just not like you. The city's gonna make you pay for that fire hydrant, ya know."

Clyde was in his customary green coveralls with *The Yard Barber* stitched across the front. He was drenched in perspiration, and his hickory-colored hair stuffed under a gray Twins baseball cap was dripping sweat down his neck. His pupils were the size of a typed period and half-moon dark areas underscored his eyes. "It's not the mowing, Becky. It's my sleep. It's hard to fiction when you ain't sleepin'."

"You mean function?"

"What?"

"Never mind. Did you know your face is twitchin'?" And your eyeballs are so small!"

"Let me take a sh . . . a . . . sh . . ."

"A shower?"

He nodded.

"Of course, Clyde. Be careful. You seem out of sorts."

After he took a shower, he laid down on the leather couch in the living room and tried to sleep. Twenty minutes later, Becky checked on him, only to discover his eyes glaring at the ceiling.

Clyde, you okay?"

He said nothing. His eyes told her he was trying, but no words escaped.

"Clyde! What's happening?"

He sat up and scanned the room. Spotting an envelope from the afternoon mail, he grabbed a pen from the kitchen drawer.

I can't talk, but I see everything clearly. My mind is fine, but I can't speak.

She read it and stared at him with deep concern and more fear than she wanted to show. Her stomach churned, and she stifled the urge to throw up. His face continued to twitch. That night, when Clyde Turrentine finally slept, he never awoke.

15

Bozeman, Montana

Bill, Henry, and Hashy were on time at the IHOP and waited for Enzo before moving into any discussion of deaths. They sat in their usual corner booth so two of them could keep an eye on anyone coming into the restaurant, and the other two could signal if anyone approached their table. The smell of yeast overlaid with coffee fumes hovered in the air.

"You think Enzo has told Sachi anything?" Henry asked.

"I hope not," Hashy replied. "We made a pact. Marriage doesn't change that."

When Enzo walked in, he hiked his bifocals up, nervously scanned the room, and hurried to their table.

"What's wrong, Enzo?"

"Something's not right. It feels like someone's watching me. I see parked cars on my street I've never seen. I mean who blacks out their windows in Montana? And I've noticed some static on my cell phone calls. We're safe, right?" he asked with little certitude.

Bill leaned into the table. "I wasn't going to mention this, since I thought I was paranoid, but there was someone at JJ asking for me. When my receptionist told the guy I wasn't there, he started asking lots of questions, and they weren't about marijuana. He didn't buy any, either. No one comes into my place and leaves without product. Now that Enzo mentioned something, it sounds like we need to be more careful."

"How can we be more careful?" Henry asked excitedly. "We don't call each other, don't text, no emails, no mail, no chat groups. Nothing. We only see each other at IHOP. BNF helped us get new identities, so what else could we do?"

"What if it's BNF showing up?" asked Enzo, drops of sweat appearing above his eyebrows in the air-conditioned restaurant.

"That's crazy," said Bill. "They have just as much to lose—"

"What if they're trying to shut us up? Tie up loose ends?" asked Henry. His questions did silence them. No one spoke for more than a minute.

"Christ!" Hashy finally said. "I've had some odd static on my cell as well. I thought it was just AT&T acting up again until I heard you guys talkin'. This is not good."

"I knew this was a mistake from the beginning," said Henry. "But BNF no longer exists, guys, so it can't be them, right?"

"Not that we know of," said Bill. "Maybe we don't meet here anymore, either. Enzo, what if we meet at your place in the mountains in a fortnight?"

The cannabis connoisseur loved to read old British novels. The other three members of the quartet took it in stride.

"That gives us enough time to tie up loose ends, get enough food and essentials to last maybe a month? My receptionist can take over for me at the shop, and you guys all have the ability to take off for a while, right?"

They all nodded.

"Enzo, you can bring Sachi if you want. How does everyone feel about the plan?"

The others sat nervously for a minute as they ran through their own implications.

Enzo said, "I can send Sachi to her mothers in Denver. I'd rather her go there than where we'll be."

"You considered what you'll tell her?" asked Hashy, her green eyes accusatory.

"Yes." He focused on a recently used ashtray in the center of the table, averting his gaze from the others, hesitating before continuing. "Our marriage . . . it's been on the rocks lately. I can say I need time and will be headed to the cabin for some head-clearing. She'll go to her mother's, for sure. I won't need to coax her."

"I'm sorry to hear that, Enzo." Bill patted Enzo's shoulder.

"It's okay. It's not over, but this is an ideal time to take a break."

"I'm in," said Hashy. "The sooner, the better. It won't take long to tie up any loose ends for me."

"Can we just go up when we're ready, Enzo? No need to wait the fourteen days, right?" Henry was eager and more than a little nervous about the sudden uptick in unusual incidents.

"Nope. You guys know where it is, and there's a key to the cabin between two bricks in the firepit behind the house."

"So, we're set?" Bill asked. They all nodded an affirmation, then paid for their breakfast and broke for their cars.

A black sedan was parked at the gas station next door. A message was sent.

16

Phoenix, Arizona

Kyle hurried into his private office when Georgina interrupted a consultation with the wife of one of his insomnia flu patients.

"Hey Marie, I've been wondering about your progress. Thanks for calling."

"I've made a few more inquiries. Found they've already been running autopsies on these patients. However, the results are considered confidential, and they're using HIPAA as a shield against disclosure." Marie's distaste of government intrusion into health care in general was evident.

"Am I about to hear a libertarian discourse?" Kyle asked.

"It's tempting, but no time. I'm working every angle I can, but I'm not the only one. On social media, there're other sleep researchers who appear to be putting the pieces together, but honestly, Kyle, even if and when we discover this is a prion disease and *if* the diagnosis is FFI, we then have to discover how it's being transmitted. That's not even addressing the cure. We're not even close to discovering a cure for prion diseases and they've been around, or should I say we've *known* about them, since 1985."

"Sounds like we have an uphill climb."

"Yes, an uphill climb on a sheet of ice. I've been running this exercise through my mind. You're sixty-one and I'm forty-seven. For argument's sake, let's say everyone in their fifties dies. Is it then over, or will those like me who turn fifty in three years then be subject to contracting InF?"

"I assume that question is rhetorical."

"Quite. Right now, this is so new there's not an ICD-10-CM code for InF yet. If there was, and if all physicians used it, the insurance companies could help us develop a large enough database so we could discover common markers besides just being middle-aged."

"Have you found any commonalities yourself yet?" asked Kyle.

"Not a single one, but I'm only considering health histories. Are they morning larks or night owls? Do they drink scotch? Are they Capricorns? We know nothing now, so we need data for the statisticians to develop some answers. I doubt we have anything close to a Gaussian distribution here. I don't think it's contagious after talking to my patients, but even that's a guess. Probably safest to have our middle-aged patients self-quarantine, but the numbers aren't high enough to force the government's hand in this, considering how they handled the coronavirus in the early stages."

"Thanks, Marie. That's what I've been telling my patients in that demographic. I've also been notifying friends and family, and unfortunately, some I've spoken with have already developed some of the symptoms."

"God help us, Kyle . . . God help us."

17

Headline news from the *Arizona Times Herald*, May 6, 2021.

If COVID did not bring enough suffering and death, the new mysterious illness known as insomnia flu is threatening to be a worthy sequel. "Little is known at this time," admits Dr. Axel Throckmorton, chief epidemiologist at Allegheny General Hospital in Pittsburgh and author of The Extramarital Disease, a retrospective glance at how new diseases have been brought to light. "We are still early in the game. Not until we are north of one thousand documented cases are we capable of making an intelligent DOD (declaration of disease)." We will have more on this critical subject in the coming days.

"Hey, boss. Getting lots of calls—"

"Yes, I'm aware, Tom. It was expected. Do you have anything *new* to report?" Jacob was on edge after he received a call at 4:30 a.m. that Sylvia had succumbed to InF during the night. "I'm sorry, Tom. Didn't mean to bark at you."

"It's okay, sir, under the circumstances." Tom was again speaking to Jacob through his partially opened office door.

Jacob always promoted an open-door policy with his team and had considered closing it this morning but decided against it, knowing some may need to talk to him about Sylvia.

"Let me know if you need anything, sir." Tom walked back to his desk.

Jacob was reflective, but to get his mind off Sylvia, he chose to think of the story instead. The piece did not surprise anyone. It was more of an uncovering of the elephant everyone knew was there. The piece Landon had written produced many more questions than answers, but he did a respectable job of laying them out in a way promoting logical thinking. Jacob was proud of that. He made a snap decision and stepped out of his office. As he stood still and gazed out over the large room, his team realized he was asking for their attention. The noise softened until the only sound was the air conditioner and the ringing of unanswered phones.

"As you all know, our beloved editor, Sylvia, passed during the night. We will announce arrangements within the next few days. You may not have all loved her, but her job was not to collect your love. Her job was to gain your respect and to put forth a product we could all be proud of. For those two jobs, I give her an A plus. We will not be able to replace her. She was one-of-a-kind in the world of editing.

"However, that was not her greatest accomplishment. She accepted me as her friend, which takes much more skill and perseverance than editing a newspaper. What we can *not* do is allow her life, memory, struggles, and death to pass without meaning or purpose.

"I have decided to create a new section in the *Arizona Times Herald*. It will focus on the medical or health topics currently impacting our lives, for good or bad. This section will be called 'Sylvia's Touch.'"

This earned a round of applause with hands moistened from wiping away tears.

After a respectful moment, Jacob continued. "The first mission of 'Sylvia's Touch' will be to investigate this insomnia flu until we have every answer needed. I believe it can be done, and I urge you to consider this challenge as one we alone are capable of winning."

This statement brought some expected furrowed brows.

"Yes, I know there are many resources available, and the experts will be searching for answers, but don't be fooled into thinking they're in a better place to forge a resolution. We will not rest until the cause is revealed and the cure is discovered. Are you with me?"

A resounding, "Yes!" echoed through the seventh floor. "Are you with Sylvia?" This time, the first floor heard it. Jacob retreated into his office to outline the game plan.

18

Bozeman, Montana

The sun disappeared over Bridger Mountain, cooling down the Montana evening. Henry shaved, mixed himself a French Connection, and packed in the bedroom twilight. He sent an email to FedEx, letting his boss know he would be taking the sick and vacation days he had earned to "discover myself" and to "come back stronger," so he could be "the best employee at FedEx."

He decided to head to Enzo's place in the morning to get a head start on the others. He could get the best room. He packed two suitcases and two large ice chests with food and drinks he would need. Two cases of Miller Lites, four bottles of Tito's vodka and mixers, two bottles of Rémy Martin, two five-gallon jugs of Sparkletts, and three bags of double-stuffed Oreos.

He packed the car with the suitcases and ice chests, then went back inside to watch an episode of *Hannibal* before he went to sleep. He guzzled the bottle of Rémy Martin to make sure he was asleep before the credits rolled. It was a fitful sleep as he dreamed of a black sedan running him down, and about a vine growing quickly, wrapping him in a vice grip, squeezing the air out of his lungs. This dream was interrupted with another dream—an explosion. The fire consumed him, but this was not a dream.

The explosion tore apart the wall between his bedroom and the kitchen, throwing burning wallpaper and drywall across his bed. Henry was enveloped in flames, his flannel pajamas ablaze, but layers of debris prevented him from escape. Fiery tentacles licked at every vulnerable appendage and orifice. He survived for fifteen seconds before his heart stopped beating for the last time. He did not hear the fire engines as they drew closer.

> #41 will not make the party tonight.
> Roger. Will send party favor.

19

The Arizona Times Herald, May 7, 2021.

The Carlotta Foundation Hospital in Topeka, Kansas has reported multiple admissions of patients with complaints of insomnia. Admission reports from 2020 revealed only two patients presenting with this complaint in the entire year, but in the first week of May, they reported eleven cases. Blood samples have shown nothing unusual, there is no genetic link, and the medication profiles show no similarities. Reports from other parts of the country are similar. Early on, the diagnosis of these unfortunate citizens has been termed insomnia flu or InF.

Phoenix, Arizona

"Jilian, before I lose my ability to speak, I need you to contact Governor Adair for me. He may want to disgust . . . *discuss* this over the phone. I'd like to submit Judge Tracy Stout . . . Judge . . ."

"Stoutmeyer. Judge Stoutmeyer."

"Yes, thank you. She would be a worthy replacement for me when I become inca . . . when I can't finish my term. I'm sure you understand my . . . you understand." Senator Bonner sat in a semi-reclined position in the white chaise lounge her staff had given her on the first anniversary of her first term. Her Persian cat jumped up and nestled on her chest.

Jilian sat in one of the Britton armchairs reserved for guests, her black hair pulled back into a ponytail. The lights were dimmed in the windowless room, hurting the press secretary's ability to raise spirits.

"Yes, Senator. Not my favorite subject, but I'm here for you. Do you think the governor will appoint Stoutmeyer on your recommendation?"

"I hope so," she said, with a greater measure of energy. This subject had raised her blood pressure each time it was broached. "I know he might want Gargs . . . no Griggs. That bastard supported Adair's brother's laws . . . in-law . . . whatever that bill was . . . I don't want . . . my work on the . . . Black Cattle . . . no Kettle Initiative to be . . . uh . . . wasted. I know the judge will carry it . . . carry on for me."

"I'll do my best. Just rest now. I'll take it from here." As she left the room, Jilian wondered how many more conversations she would have with her friend. The senator chose her from a pool of seventy-five applicants after she had won her first term, and for the last six years had treated her like the sister she never had. She was determined to convince the governor that the judge would be her best replacement. She hurried down the hall toward her office but was interrupted by her assistant.

"Ms. Quito, have you seen the latest death toll numbers for Arizona?" She was handing her a folder as she spoke.

"Thanks, Elizabeth."

"I've also included stats for all fifty states. I think you'll spot some interesting data."

Jilian entered her office and laid out the sheets before her.

Arizona InF Deaths	428 (one for every 17,023 citizens)
% of InF deaths age 50-59	98.7% (one per 2026)
All others	1.3%

She noticed the outliers and thought she might mention it to the senator. She then compared Arizona to the other states, and all revealed virtually the same numbers. One out of every 2,000 in the 50-59 age group were dying from InF. Every state was in the same range.

She picked up the phone and punched the button for Governor Adair's office.

"Hey Brenda, this is Jilian."

"Oh, hey Jill. How's our senator doing? I've been praying for her."

"Not well, I'm afraid."

"I'm so sorry to hear that."

"Yeah, this is tough, and I hate bringing this up, but I fear she won't be with us much longer. She would like Governor Adair to consider Judge Stoutmeyer to finish her term."

Brenda was silent for a moment, then said, "Oh, of course! I'll be sure to get him the message, but I must make sure the timing is right. It's a rather morose message, and I can't pass that on just before he meets with someone, and he has meetings all day. It might take a few days before he can give this his attention."

"That's fine, but please don't forget. Can you consider it her dying wish?"

"Don't play that game, Jilian. I told you I'd give him the message. Give the senator my best and tell her the governor is pulling for her." *Click.*

Taken aback at Brenda's abrupt conversation, she wondered if she should tell the senator. She decided not to mention anything, since the senator was so sick.

20

"Sir, you can't bring that in here."

Bryce Davidson stared at the theater cashier as if she had three heads, two of which swiveled. "I have a permit, miss, and I can take Mr. Hobbs anywhere I goddamn want."

Slightly amused, but more than slightly perturbed, the cashier said, "You seriously call your gun Mr. Hobbs?"

He swiveled his own head in her direction. "I call my other gun Mr. Bobblehead."

At that, she stood up in the booth, cupped hands over her mouth and yelled, "Guards!" When she turned around, Davidson was gone. He had ducked into the shoe store next to the movie theater and hid behind the Cole Hahn display. He had been through multiple bypass surgeries and knew he would not live to be a hundred like his grandfather.

And now, sleep evaded him. "What else you got for me, God?" he yelled through the stupors he experienced as he moved between wakefulness and sleep. It was difficult enough to navigate the transition from waking systems to those turned off when crossing the sensitive sheen of resistance into the first stage of sleep. It became even more strained when Davidson's eyes would not close, and his heart rate would rise. This became his new normal, and he did not like it.

That night, as he made his way home after ensuring the theater guards had given up the search, he reflected on the past two months. Losing weight was okay as he had plenty to lose, but he was slowly losing the ability to communicate. He could yell at his Red Sox on television, but then no one could judge his ability to make sense. He even made no sense to himself. He sat down at the table in his breakfast nook and peered into a silver pitcher, which showed a hazy reflection of his aging face. He pulled Mr. Hobbs's trigger.

21

"Dr. Hunter? Dr. Jimmerson is here."

"Please show her in. This must be important."

Marie slid through the door, her light feet soundless on his WPC flooring. He pointed to the Castor lounge chair he had added for guests. "Have a seat! To what do I owe the pleasure?" He steepled his fingers.

She shed her clinic jacket to reveal a one-piece floral dress, loosely tied at the waist. "I need your help. You're friends with Jacob Potter at the *Arizona Times Herald*?"

He leaned back in his chair and folded his hands behind his head. "We play golf together. Actually, *he* plays. I mostly thrash and weep, generally making a fool of myself. But yeah, our wives are friends from college, so we get together for dinner maybe . . . once a month? What's up?"

"I can't get any traction with the Arizona medical board. They say a prion disease is out of the question, but I see too many signs. I know Jacob isn't afraid of the establishment and likes to ruffle some feathers. You think you could get him to activate his radar on this?"

"First, tell me more about our medical board. I've stayed out of politics. The one guy I know took seven times to pass the boards, so I don't give them much credit. It wouldn't take much to do an autopsy and study the brain tissue, would it?"

"Neither of us are coroners, Kyle . . . or neurosurgeons, so this is out of our league. But they keep saying it's encephalitis, and they're discovering it's viral-related, but there's no cause and effect here. I've been doing more research on prions, and they can make a cell more susceptible to invasion by a virus. Encephalitis is one of the hallmarks of fatal familial insomnia. Remember, FFI?"

Kyle nodded.

"I think they're trying to pass these off as COVID deaths . . . or at least most of them. I suspect we have many more InF deaths than we know."

"Geez, Marie. You're sounding like a conspiracy theorist now." He smiled.

"Will you ask Jacob or not?" She sat straighter in her chair and stiffened her back. Her fair skin pinked up quickly.

Kyle's blue eyes narrowed as he leaned forward in his chair, placed one hand on the desk in front of him and overlayed it with the second. "Now, now, Marie. Don't get worked up. I'm on your side, and yes, I will speak with Jacob. He's always hunting for stories, so it won't be awkward at all."

"Why don't you call him right now?" she asked, arching her back in a challenging pose.

"Well, why not?" He reached over to pick up his cell phone and searched for Jacob, then punched the number, putting it on speaker. Marie settled back into her chair and the temporary flush faded.

"You've reached Jacob Potter. I'm out walking my donkey, but as soon as I get my ass back in, I'll call you back. Leave me a message."

"Very funny, Jacob. Hey, I've got Dr. Marie Jimmerson here. She's a sleep medicine physician with a history of epidemiological sleep research as well. She's developed an interesting theory on these insomnia flu victims. Give me a call if you want to discuss it with her. I think it would be worth investigating. Tell Wendy hello for me, and I hope you get your ass back in soon. Someone as old as you should take it easy in the heat." He ended the call, then glanced at Marie with a satisfied expression.

"Think he'll call back?" Marie asked, as she stood and angled toward the door.

"I'm sure he will." His cell began playing John Fogerty's "Headlines."

"Told you he'd call."

Marie eagerly walked back to the chair and sat down. Kyle put it on speaker and said, "Jacob! Thanks for calling back. You caught Dr. Jimmerson while she was still here. You're on speaker."

"Hello, Dr. Jimmerson. Nice to virtually meet you." Jacob's tone was tinged with excitement.

"Please, call me Marie." She unveiled a breathy, nuanced voice, which betrayed a tone of self-assurance.

"Done. So, Marie, what have you got for me?"

"I'm not a conspiracy theorist as Dr. Hunter here inferred—"

"No comment," said Kyle.

"I've read in one of your editorials that you feel the number of COVID deaths has been inflated."

"We haven't exactly buried those opinions."

"I think there are more than the reported one out of every two thousand in their fifties dying of the insomnia flu also. I think it's being underreported."

"Do you have any proof?" Jacob's voice betrayed his excitement.

"Not what you would classify as proof, but I think I can get you to believe we need to investigate this closer."

"Go on."

"Have you had a chance to study the age demographics of COVID deaths?"

"Well, yes, I have."

"I read your paper every day."

"Thank you. There's at least one reader."

"I've read it daily, and you gloss over the deaths by age, but I have yet to see you publish any number over a six-month period, for example."

"You're about to tell me you've done this for us." It sounded like a statement and a question.

"Exactly. You can run these numbers yourself, but why would we have thirty-four percent of all COVID deaths occurring in people in their fifties, but only twelve percent of these deaths in people in their sixties?"

"If this is about math, I need to get my calculator out or call my eight-year-old grandson into the office. But I agree, so far it sounds odd."

"And people in their forties only make up four percent of all COVID deaths."

"Okay, this doesn't add up."

"No, it doesn't. Were you aware hospitals are paid twenty percent more if a patient is diagnosed with COVID instead of pneumonia? And if they're put on a ventilator, they get paid so much that hospitals are now having ethics battles in their board rooms." Kyle nodded at Marie's statement, having read the statistics himself.

"So, I guess you're saying we have many more dying from this insomnia flu than we think?"

"Far more," she said emphatically, "but that's not all."

"I'm still taking notes."

"I don't think this is any type of flu. I know they're calling it encephalitis that comes from a virus, but I think it's a prion disease and not a virus at all."

"Please spell that disease for me."

"P.R.I.O.N."

"Got it. If we print something about a disease, we damn well better spell it right."

"We have a few challenges, though.

"Don't we all."

"As far as we know, prion diseases that affect humans aren't transmissible through contact or aerosols, so the rate of infection is not what we would expect."

"And?"

"If we don't know how it's transmitted, we don't know how many will or could contract it, and on top of that, we don't know how to mount a defense."

"Sounds like you read the *Arizona Times Herald* this morning."

Marie eyed Kyle quizzically. "No, I usually read it after work, but I plan on reading it when I get back to my office now that you've piqued my interest. Are you already investigating this?"

"Our managing editor, Sylvia Witherspoon, died last night, and we're fairly sure it was the insomnia flu, or whatever we should be calling it. We've been ready to publish a piece for the last week. Just waiting for the right time."

"I'm so sorry. I don't mean to be insensitive, but could you tell me how long she had been having any symptoms?"

"That's not being insensitive. You'd make a good reporter. If you ever want to give up that doctor gig, let me know."

"I appreciate the compliment, but I can't spell . . . well, anything but prion."

"From what everyone knows, I would say she's had some symptoms for maybe two months, not much longer."

Marie sighed. "This is what I've been seeing in my own patient base as well. In classical FFI, we see—"

"FFI?" Jacob asked.

"Sorry. Fatal familial insomnia. In most cases, we see one to two years of struggling before they succumb in known cases of FFI. This must be a new subtype."

"It appears I'll need to do some research on this FFI, but I need some reassurance that there's a high probability this is what we're seeing before I commit substantial resources."

"Even with the time differential we're seeing between onset of symptoms and death, I still give it an eighty-percent chance we're seeing at least a strain of FFI."

"Kyle, do you vouch for our Dr. Jimmerson?"

"Yes, I do. She's no conspiracy theorist."

22

Bozeman, Montana

Enzo Caputo felt both exhilarated and anxious. As he expected, Sachi decided to stay with her mother. He did still love her, even with their recent rifts.

He drove north toward the cabin he bought with the money BNH paid him for his work in Verona. They appropriated his research and morphed it into an agent for death, but they paid him handsomely for it. The guilt he felt after maneuvering around his friends and coworkers was something he lived with daily. His property was bought with blood money, but twenty years ago, his affections were influenced by the zero-population growth movement that grew from Dr. Paul Ehrlich's *The Population Bomb*. Now, he just wanted to forget. Forget that he stole into his father's lab every night to test his theories. Forget that he connected online with Dietrich Monnag. Forget that he agreed to help BNH. But he knew he would not be allowed to forget.

He packed his Lexus for a six-week stay at his own Camp Caputo. It was only a cabin, but growing up, he had been jealous of friends who went to camp during the Venetian summers while he was going to summer school. Both of his parents felt he could get ahead this way, but they were not alive, and he could now go to camp anytime he wanted.

His drive was not without angst, gazing repeatedly into his rearview mirror for any sign of his imagined opposition. Ahead, as Bridger Mountain rose into the skyline, he envisioned machine-toting mercenaries skiing down the snowless slopes toward him.

Enzo was the shortest of their quartet, and when he drove solo, he would place a back cushion under his butt so his head would rise above steering wheel height. His unshaven, black, two-day beard chaffed his neck as he swiveled side to side, expecting at any moment a cadre of motorcycles with headless riders to float by and toss burning embers through his window. He checked his phone to see if Sachi had tried to contact him, knowing he would see no evidence. He turned on 102.9 FM KSCY and Keith Urban was singing, "Better Life." At least it kept his mind off Sachi and the memories he ached to forget.

It would be a two-hour drive to Camp Caputo, and he wondered if anyone would beat him there. He loved the drive, particularly this time of year when the journey was less treacherous, but he missed the calving sheets of snow in the midday sun as the Bridger mountains shed their layers like a child throwing off unwanted covers. He decided to return in the fall to enjoy the show and marvel at the fresh blanket of purity that amazed him every year. Like clockwork, this area hibernated under a white bedspread until spring brought enough warmth to wake up the sleeping mountain range.

He came to the familiar wildlife guard he placed in the road to keep deer out of his fenced-in property and rounded the corner. He expected to see his shuddered windows from the winter before, but he skidded to a halt. His tires threw up dust and gravel to create a temporary envelope of brown haze. When it cleared, he got a better picture of the body suspended from the crossbeam on his front porch. The limp, lifeless body of Hashtag "Hashy" Wareness hung from a rope, head hanging over the noose that suffocated the life out of her. It took him a few seconds to recover from the shock, and when he did, he put his Lexus into reverse and backed up fifty feet, then spun around and headed back down the mountain. He drove frantically for a mile, then slowed and stopped, angling off the road.

His mind raced, but he soon turned his attention to his options. His analytic mind went into hyperdrive. The killer, or killers, could still be there. It had to be murder because there was no stool kicked to the side. It was highly likely they saw him, if they were there, and heard his car. But since no one showed themselves, maybe they were no longer there. If he went back and there were no threats of danger, what would he then do?

Get her body down? It was a murder scene.

Call the police? Could they be trusted?

If someone saw him drive away, it would appear as if he either killed her or left a crime scene without calling the police.

This was a no-win situation for Enzo Caputo. He considered calling Bill or Henry but knew that would be foolish. He considered driving to Sachi's mother's house but knew it could endanger them. He decided he would drive to a hotel nearby and use a payphone, wondering if those were still around—maybe a burner phone to call Bill and Henry. He started the car again and drove back down the mountain, now able to mourn Hashy properly.

23

Phoenix, Arizona

"Danny, I know you haven't heard of FFI, but I've been doing some research over the weekend, and I think this is what we're seeing with this insomnia flu epidemic." Jacob had called his executive editor into his office and handed him a manila envelope. "Have a seat. This will take a few minutes. I've put together the start of a lead story for 'Sylvia's Touch' on Sunday, but I need you and the writers to flesh this out. We have a local source who I prefer not to reveal right now. She introduced the possibility of FFI, which stands for fatal familial insomnia." He sounded the words out carefully.

Danny sat on the couch Jacob used as a bed when he was up late resolving loose ends or when he and Wendy were not in the mood to sleep together. He pulled the material out of the envelope and quickly scanned the contents. "What's this article on sleeping sickness?"

Jacob grinned. "I traveled down some interesting rabbit trails and stumbled over that story. I don't know how many are familiar with this since it was a century ago, but in the winter of 1916-17, in the middle of World War I, this sleeping sickness killed over a million people."

"That's news to me," said Danny. If Danny were to choose between bouts of food poisoning and learning history, he would be throwing up with regularity.

"The 1918 Spanish influenza pandemic also overshadowed sleeping sickness, so it was largely ignored. The real name for it is encephalitis lethargica—"

"Wait a second. Is that in these documents somewhere?"

"Yes, but the important part is that many of the symptoms were the same as what we're seeing with this current insomnia flu. I don't want COVID to keep our attention off this flu like the big war did to sleeping sickness." Jacob sat on the edge of his desk as they talked. "One thing that stood out to me; there is no evidence of this in any other country, not even Mexico or Canada. Everywhere I searched, there were reports relating to the insomnia flu in every area of the U.S., but not a single mention outside the States. It's different from sleeping sickness because that was passed to citizens in many countries."

Danny rubbed the back of his neck. "You're telling me this doesn't appear to be contagious? We suspected it wasn't, but it's sounding like there is no question now."

"Correct. And what this also means is that it's highly likely this insomnia flu was foisted on our country by either a monumental mistake or by a group of miscreants bent on eliminating a subset of our society. I don't know which would be worse."

Danny took notes on the outside of the envelope. Raising his eyes to address Jacob, he said, "Oh, if you haven't heard, Ted, down in the mailroom, is having some of the same symptoms Sylvia was having. I know everyone here is hypersensitive to this after what happened to Sylvia. Some may have psychosomatic responses, but

Ted's not like that, or at least the Ted I know isn't."

Jacob shook his head slowly. "Put both Kira and Sawyer on this. I want our best investigators working on it."

Danny stopped writing. "So, take them off—"

"I said I want Kira and Sawyer. Whatever you have to do to get that done is fine with me."

"Yes sir," he said resignedly. "You listed five directives you want us to attack. Can we discuss those quickly so I can be sure we're on the same page?"

"Certainly," Jacob said, as he walked around his desk to sit in his chair.

Danny found the sheet in the envelope and extracted it. "First, research if there is a disproportionate number of people in their fifties being diagnosed with the coronavirus. I understand the reason for that one. Second, see if the insomnia flu is being missed in other age groups. I assume this is to see if the authorities are being myopic?"

Jacob nodded. "We have to be missing some. Doesn't make sense to be restricted to people in their fifties."

"Check. Third, scout for trends—run analytics. Do we use our team for this, or do you want me to outsource it?"

"Best we outsource. I like our people, but the Mayweather Group out of Seattle is who I've used for other projects and they're unbelievably insightful—very thorough. And perhaps most important, they're loyal. They won't sell what they learn to the highest bidder."

"Got it," Danny said. "Fourth, investigate the Zero Population Group. Can you give me some context here?"

"We received an anonymous tip that emphatically stated the ZPG organization is behind the insomnia flu. We assumed it was some crackpot and filed it away, but it's worth considering."

"That's a stretch, but we'll check it out. Fifth, try to disprove this is FFI. I think you've provided some material for us to read, so I'll let you know if we have any questions on that one later. Is there anything else you need us to do?"

"Yes. Discover a cure." Jacob's expression was serious.

"I assume the medical community is working that angle, but if we run across a cure, you'll be the first to know."

Danny strode to his office and texted Sawyer and Kira to hand off their projects to their subs and meet him in his office stat.

At a quarter to three, Kira showed up at Danny's office. She leaned a shamrock-colored umbrella in the corner and sat in a highbacked chair situated a few feet in front of Danny's desk. She swept her long, unbound caramel hair over her shoulders, revealing a slender neck circled by a silver chain that hung just above a sky-blue cotton knit polo shirt. "What's up, Danny?"

"Is it raining out there?"

"Just a threat. I like to be prepared."

"You would've made a good Boy Scout. I'm putting you two on the insomnia flu. We're going all out on this, and Jacob's given us carte blanche to go as deep and wide as we can. It's almost personal with him. Guess Sylvia's death hit him harder than I thought."

"He didn't take it well," Kira said. "They were very close. Did you know Sylvia introduced Jacob to Wendy?"

"No, I didn't."

Be there in 7

They both glanced at their phones.

"Sawyer's almost here so I'll wait to go into more detail when he gets here," said Danny. "How's the boyfriend?"

Kira narrowed her eyes and adjusted herself in the chair. The fact he smelled of tobacco and after shave that would draw an army of ants only added to her disgust of her immediate boss.

"His name is Carter and he's fine."

Kira had noticed Danny ogling her uncomfortably in the past, almost to the extent that she would report his behavior, but it never became more than that.

"So, you're still together?" Danny probed.

"What's this all about, Danny?"

"Just making conversation, Kira. Nothing else."

"OK, how's Debra?" she asked. She knew they were not doing well and wanted to get the subject off her.

"Ouch. Well, we're getting divorced." He glanced at Kira, expecting a response, but none came. She was not keen on continuing the trajectory of the conversation.

"I'll be right back," she said, standing and turning toward the door. "I need to get my notebook. I get the feeling we'll be on this assignment for a while, and I need to get my thoughts organized." Walking out the door, she felt his eyes on her and shivered.

Ten minutes after she had left, she walked back in behind Sawyer.

"Morning, Danny!" he said as they found seats in front of Danny's desk. Kira felt better with reinforcements.

"Thanks for coming," Danny said.

"Kira filled me in a little," Sawyer said, "so you can pick up where you left off with her."

Kira hid her smirk. *Yeah—start with your divorce, Napoleon.*

"Great," Danny replied. "I'll get right to it." For the next thirty minutes, he explained the directives Jacob had relayed, outlined a game plan, and assigned duties to Sawyer and Kira. He gave the insomnia flu demographics and Zero Population Group to Sawyer, FFI to Kira, and said he would get with the Mayweather Group to run some analytics.

"When you say *carte blanche*, Danny," Sawyer said, "is there an expense limit?"

"Nothing's in stone, but let's say if any item is over a thousand, I need to approve. That's until further notice."

They both nodded and left the office. This time, Kira led.

24

The reception room was packed by the time Kyle arrived. Nan greeted him at the door.

"You've got a waiting room full of insomniacs, Dr. Hunter. Most of them said they weren't sleeping anyway, so they decided to show up. They don't mind waiting because they've established somewhat of a camaraderie out there."

"How do they know this isn't contagious? How do *we* know this isn't contagious?"

"Everyone's wearing masks, so I'm sure they're not worried."

Kyle had an idea. He peered through the window, taking care not to be seen, and as expected, saw a roomful of middle-aged men and women, evenly divided by sex. They appeared to be comparing notes. Some were further along the symptom pathway than others and had more stories to tell. None, it appeared, had lost the ability to speak, which Kyle determined to be the final symptom before death. This was corroborated by Dr. Marie Jimmerson.

"Nan, we have a significant database. Can you run a list of every patient in their fifties?"

"Of course. It will take me a few minutes."

Kyle picked up the phone and called Marie's office.

"She's with a patient right now. May I leave her a message?"

"Yes, please. I have an idea on learning what started this new flu epidemic."

"Wow. I'm sure she'll want to hear about this. Let me see if I can pull her—"

"No, no. Just have her call when she gets a chance. I still have some details to work out."

Nan returned with an eight-page printed list. "We have three hundred and fifty-six active patients in their fifties."

"Great. Can you get your daughter? She's still searching for a job, right?"

"Yes, she is," Nan said.

"Please get her to call each one or text—actually both—and ask if they can come to a town hall meeting at the YMCA on Lebanon at seven o'clock on the fourteenth. The topic will be the insomnia flu, what we know, and what we're working on. They don't need to RSVP . . . just come if you can. Think she can do that?"

"Might take a few days, but—"

"That's why I said the fourteenth. If she starts right now, she's got plenty of time to get it done. The Y hasn't opened back up, but I know the city manager. He'll let us use it, but I need a week to get everything set up."

"What do you have in mind?" Nan asked.

"Having a discussion with some talking points and a survey to start things off. It could give us some insight and might uncover a few pearls."

"I hope you're right. They could keep you there all night. You know they can't sleep."

"Ha-ha."

"Okay, I'll get Laura on that immediately."

"You could start with who we have in the waiting room right now."

For the next hour, Kyle let his two physician assistants see his patients. They had been seeing these insomniacs for weeks now and they knew what to ask, what to check, how to observe, and what to suggest. He created a list of questions and some open-ended discussion points that he would moderate at the YMCA event.

The next day in the late afternoon, Georgina knocked on Kyle's door. He recognized her painful gait as she traveled the fifty feet between her desk and his door. "Come in, Georgina!"

"How'd you know it was me?" she asked, as she opened the door.

"I recognized your knock."

"Oh . . . well, I wanted you to know that the phone hasn't stopped ringing about your party."

Kyle groaned under his strained smile. "It's not a party, Georgina, but that's good to hear."

25

"Brenda, has the governor made a decision? The senator may not last until tomorrow." Jilian wiped her tears, smudging newly applied makeup as she spoke. Her eyes were going on three days of redness and swelling, her fingernails chewed and worn. Her angular chin showed recent stress wrinkles, but one could still see strong evidence of an aging porcelain face. Senator Bonner could no longer talk, using a notepad to communicate, and was hallucinating. There were tigers in her room one minute and wasps the next. It took all of Jilian's fortitude to prevent her from breaking down in her presence. Seeing an intelligent, vivacious, dogmatic, charismatic senator and friend reduced to this in the span of six months tore her apart. She often went into the bathroom, turned on the sink and let it all go, the kaleidoscope of emotions cascading in layers as she reminisced on the sixteen years she had spent at her side.

"The governor's been extremely busy, Jilian. I've tried to—"

"Dammit, Brenda! Why are you stonewalling us? She's given her life to this office and championed almost every cause the governor's asked for. How can you do this?" She tried to stay strong and push the emotions down, but the struggle was transparent to Brenda.

"Jilian, I am deeply sorry. My hands are tied." Although the governor and senator had allegiances to different parties, they managed to work together for the good of Arizona, forging a relationship, which was lauded, incredibly, by the typically caustic press. During recent months, however, both Senator Bonner and Jilian had noticed a chasm slowly opening. Calls were not returned, rumors of tension drew life, and an associate judge on the Arizona Supreme Court was released of duties by Governor Adair. The judge was coming up for reelection, but in an unprecedented move, he used his powers to shed a vocal opponent of police corruption. "I just can't give you the assurance you seek. The governor is not ready to make a decision."

"You can tell the governor to go to hell!" Jilian hit the red button on her cell to end the call, channeling 1988 when she could slam the phone down and feel more satisfaction.

She burst from her private office on the second floor inside the senator's home and went downstairs to check on her.

The senator had lost fifty-five pounds in the last ninety days and appeared so emaciated sitting at her desk that Jilian could see skin slipping away from her right arm, exposing bone. Her nurse stood by, waiting on any request the senator had, but none came. Jilian stood in awe of the senator's perseverance. She never heard her complain about her sickness, the pain she felt, or her inability to cook a meal or finish a thought. She did not notice Jilian enter the room.

She had finished updating her will earlier in the day and her attorney came by to make it legal. She wrote a goodbye letter to the people she had served and asked Jilian not to read it until she was eulogized.

She wrote she had, ". . . made peace with my enemies . . . I assure you I'll be observing you from beyond the grave to make sure you continue to fight the good fight."

That night, lying awake as Phoenix slept, the heart she used to care for so many beat one last time.

26

Bozeman, Montana

Enzo continued to wrestle with a decision on where to go after seeing Hashy's body swaying under the awning at his cabin. It was a beautiful day in Bozeman, but when he thought back, he only saw a dark, grisly, evil afternoon. Getting over the shock proved more troublesome than he had expected, but he hoped a night of sleep in room number 146 of the Fordham Motel would prove to be medicinal. There was no pay phone, and he did not want to risk going out to buy a burner phone, so he gave up his thought to contact Bill or Henry for now.

His SUV was still packed with enough food and drink for weeks in the cabin, so he decided to sleep before making plans. With the sheer curtains and the interstate less than one hundred feet from his room, he pulled out his eye mask and ear plugs from his duffle bag first. He was hungry, so he ordered a pan pizza from Domino's. It took over an hour to arrive, but it was consumed, along with half a dozen Miller Lites in twenty minutes. He passed out soon after that.

He awoke the next morning, lips pasted together better than most sealed envelopes, and contemplated his next move. Hashy was dead and he did not know the health of Bill or Henry. He decided to head for Bill's home, trusting his leadership skills over Henry's insecurity. He packed and placed his bag in the Lexus, then decided to right a wrong. He trudged down what had been a navigable sidewalk in previous decades to the motel's front desk to let the proprietor know the hot water was not functional in room 146 and there was only one towel. Years ago, Enzo had developed a routine of laying a towel on the floor and using the other to dry off. The absence of a floor towel left him feeling defiled.

After he had his say with the dispassionate manager, he nervously scurried back toward his car, checked Waze to locate Bill's home, then started or attempted to start the SUV. The explosion caused by eighty pounds of bomb grade fertilizer, sixty gallons of propane, and a detonator under the vehicle, ripped through the wall of 146. One car door landed in front of the vending machine and a wheel was thrown two hundred feet. Drapes opened in 152 and 138 as a tire rolled down Highway 86.

Enzo never made it to Bill's house; he would never see the Caputo cabin again. In making some poor decisions, Enzo would never again fear the unknown.

27

Phoenix, Arizona

"I know, Tom. I know."

Three rapid knocks on his door interrupted his thoughts. "Yes?"

The door opened, and Cameron stepped halfway through. "Mr. Potter, there's a woman named Jilian Quito on the line. She was Senator Bonner's communications director, and she has some information she thinks you could use."

"I'll take it in here."

"Line three," he said, as the door closed.

"Want me to leave or stay?" Tom asked.

"Might be best if I took this alone."

Tom left to check on Ted.

"Ms. Quito, this is Jacob Potter. I was so sorry to hear of the senator's death. She was one of my heroes."

"Mine as well, Mr. Potter. May I speak off the record?"

"What if I made you an unnamed source?" Jacob asked.

"That will be fine, but when you hear what I have to say, I doubt you'll be printing anything soon. It's going to take some research on your part."

"I'm listening. This conversation is private, secure, and is not being recorded." The "secure" part was something he was fond of saying, though he knew there was little truth to it.

"The senator always trusted you. It's one reason I've contacted you and not the police." She left the sentence dangling as she waited for a rejoinder.

"Go on," he said.

"She left something for me to open after her death. Have you heard of the Klavian Triumvirate?"

"No, I haven't, but I'll know more soon," Jacob said.

"Her note says the only other person in her circle of knowledge is Judge Tracy Stoutmeyer. She also knows about the Triumvirate."

"Not much of a circle, but I'm familiar with the judge. She's good people."

"Yes, she is, but I don't think the governor appreciates that fact. She also mentions in the note that the Klavian Triumvirate consists of three influential men with loose ties to the Zero Population Group. She thinks a splinter group formed twenty-five years ago that wasn't satisfied with the ZPG's agenda because it only encouraged zero population growth. This group wanted to force the issue. She had reason to believe they're behind this new insomnia flu."

"I don't mean to sound negativistic, but from what I know about this so far . . . victims lose some control of their thoughts, hallucinate, and—"

"The senator was of sound mind until the end." Jilian's tenor had morphed into a higher, forceful, faster pitch. "I know where you're going with this, but you're wrong. She'd been working on this for months. It was not contrived by a demented mind!"

"I'm sorry, but I had to ask. Did she speculate on the identities of the three men?"

Jilian relaxed her tone but hesitated before answering. "She said . . . that Governor Adair was one of them."

"Did she have proof?" Jacob asked with increased intensity. "She and the governor didn't play in the same sandbox, so we would need incontrovertible truth."

"No proof, I'm afraid. The Triumvirate is very well insulated and—"

"Would you be willing to share the note the senator left?"

"I would consider it. Let me think on that. By the way, Senator Bonner had someone on the inside. Kevin Sandam. He worked to within a few layers of Adair, but he disappeared two weeks ago. We can't locate him. His wife is a daily thorn to the police. She's become fond of making a scene. The problem is . . ."

"Yes?"

"Adair and the police chief, Montgomery, play racquetball together. They were college buddies. Both went to Princeton in the seventies."

"Are you safe, Miss Quito?"

"Right now, I don't care. If that bastard is responsible for killing the senator and thousands, maybe millions of others, my safety is secondary. I'm counting on your organization to bring justice for those who have died and—"

"I appreciate your candor and even more your passion, but we are a newspaper, and—"

"We can't trust the police. If you won't help, I'll call—"

"Wait." Jacob stopped her. "I didn't say we wouldn't help, but we have our limitations. We don't carry firearms, and we own no bullet-proof vests. Our bullets consist of the written word and research provides our gun sights. I get to pull the trigger and we will not fail you, Miss Quito. I have personal reasons for pursuing this as well. Can we work together?"

"Thank you, Mr. Potter. The senator was right about you."

After hanging up, Jacob buzzed Danny into his office. "We've got work to do, Danny. You've got Kira and Sawyer working the I.F. case, but the road took a ninety-degree turn. I need all hands on the wheel, to mix a few metaphors. You haven't heard of the Klavian Triumvirate, have you?"

"Doesn't ring a smoking gun." Danny grinned.

"Anyway, I've heard from a reputable source that a group of three influential men may be responsible for creating this new flu. We can't play our hand yet, but Governor Adair might be one of them. I need your team to dig into his past. Go back thirty years and investigate any connection you can uncover to the Zero Population Group."

Danny typed notes on his iPad.

"We also have a missing person who could be linked as well. Name is Kevin Sandam. Went missing about two weeks ago. You can spot his wife at the police station most days, I'm told, and she should be cooperative with anyone offering help. Finally, as an FYI, it's believed the three men were the head of a group that branched off the ZPG, and the name could be the Klavian Triumvirate. Shouldn't be difficult to track down but be careful. The police chief Montgomery might have a history with the group."

"Geez, Jacob. You're sure we shouldn't get the Feds involved?"

"We might not have any choice, but my fear is that their presence would drive the group so far underground they might shake hands with the devil. We need to be invisible, and we're better at that than the guys with dark suits and indoor sunglasses."

28

"Ted shouldn't be here today." Oleta from the mailroom stood in front of Danny's desk and pleaded with him. "He's really sick, Mr. King, but he won' go home. He saying his eyebrows on fire and Ginsburg turn his underwear into mashed potatoes."

"Justice Ginsburg?" Danny responded with less concern than Oleta hoped for.

"How I know? He hallucinating. I no stick around to ask details. We told him go home, but he say if he leaves, he get fired. You no fire him, would you, Mr. King?"

Sawyer and Kira were at his door now and had been listening to the conversation. "Oleta, please get security, and see if they can either escort him home or to the hospital. We have a newspaper to run, and I've got work to do. Report back to me with the decision on Ted. You're dismissed."

Oleta stared at him for a few seconds, then whirled and brushed by Sawyer as she muttered some expletives in Spanish on her way out.

"I hope you have something we can run with," Danny said to Sawyer and Kira as they slid into the room and took seats.

"What was *that* about?" asked Kira.

"Ted down in the mailroom is starting to show symptoms, so I sent him home."

"That's good," Kira said. She crossed her legs and flicked a loose strand of hair over her left shoulder. "I'll let Sawyer go first. What I found out will require some heavy decision-making."

Sawyer wore his usual khaki's. His gray T-shirt revealed a ring of sweat at the collar, and he removed a wrinkled cobalt linen blazer as he spoke. "First, I contacted the Mayweather Group, and gave them their marching orders. They said the analytics you asked for should be ready by tomorrow. The other assignment you gave me was the ZPG. I was to search for any connection to Governor Adair or Montgomery. As a primer, the Zero Population Group campaign started in the '60s, but the name fell out of favor in the latter part of the century, so in 2002, they changed their name to *Population Connection*. There were many iterations to their web site, and after I scrubbed the existing one to discover anything on Adair or Montgomery, I gave up and used the Wayback Machine to see what I could dig up."

Danny had begun taking notes, but glanced up and asked, "So, what's the Wayback Machine?"

"It's quite useful. What's funny is *that* site also changed to Archive.org. You can plug in a website, and it'll show you its appearance in a specific year. I did turn up in a 1998 iteration an editorial that referenced a splinter group that was more radical. They saw that the ZPG was attempting to become more mainstream, because they were increasingly being seen as an extremist group, and the splinter group wanted no part of the transformation."

"Can you get me a copy of the editorial?" asked Danny.

"It's already in your in box. The editorial went on to say,

although the ZPG never intended to advocate for zero people, just zero growth, a name change was coming, even though it didn't occur for another four years. Unfortunately, it didn't name anyone specifically as part of the splinter group, so I researched the name of the editor—a Banford June—but he died in a hunting accident six years ago. I would scrub the emails from the current site and send messages asking for information but am afraid that could get into the wrong hands, so I'll be trying to make some calls over the next few days."

Danny glanced up again. "You made the right decision, but I'd rather you hold off on any more communication with them at all. Anyone could be involved. I assume you also checked our archives here?"

"That was my first focus. We wrote many articles on the ZPG in the last half century, but only one after they changed their name. We never wrote anything on a splinter group. Not sure how that was missed. That's all I've got for now. Kira?"

She had also been in the triple-digit heat, but her azure skirt and jacquard off-the-shoulder blouse contrasted starkly with Sawyer's disheveled appearance. "My assignment was to uncover as much information about the insomnia flu as I could. I started by reading *The Family That Couldn't Sleep* by D.T. Max. Then I ran a Cochrane review of articles that had been published since he did his research. I won't bore you with details—just the facts we need to move this along. Assuming what we're seeing is a version of FFI—fatal familial insomnia—we know it's a prion disease and we know they can occur sporadically, through contagious routes, or genetically, which is the most common . . . although with the numbers we're seeing with the insomnia flu, that may no longer be the case—"

"Wait," Danny said. "Remind me what a prion disease is."

"Sorry. Prions, or let's say *bad* prions, are misfolded proteins, and like your socks, you don't want your proteins folded incorrectly. In genetic cases, a mutation causes a defect in the makeup of the protein that causes it to fold clumsily, and when it touches another protein, kinda like catching somebody's yawn, it becomes misfolded as well, and a chain reaction ensues. In sporadic cases, like drawing a straight flush in five-card draw, a protein gets unlucky and folds like a limp dollar bill—"

"A straight flush is unlucky?" Sawyer asked, fanning himself with a magazine.

"It is when you go all in, and the guy across the table from you displays a royal flush. There's one disease in sheep that's been around since 1732 called scrapie—they call it that because when infected, the sheep scrape off their fleeces against rocks or trees. It's believed to be caused by prions and can be transmitted either vertically or horizontally. Now before you ask, that means we can pass it to an offspring, which is the vertical track, or a sheep can pass it to another sheep, which is the horizontal track. But there's no evidence it can be transmitted to a human."

"At least not yet," Danny said.

"Correct. Fun fact. In my research, I discovered that sheep are the only animals in the animal kingdom that depend on humans to live."

"Maybe they've found a way to get back at us for that," smirked Sawyer.

"As I mentioned, the last method for contracting a prion disease is through a contagious and infectious channel. In a prion disease like Kuru, a misfolded protein—"

"What the hell is Kuru?" Danny blurted. "Sounds like a pygmy kangaroo."

Kira rolled her eyes and continued. "It's another prion disease they found in the Fore tribe of Papua New Guinea. They cannibalized their dead, eating the brain tissue. That's what spread the disease. This is the communicable . . . or infectious method, and even though there has never been any evidence of prions being transmitted through air-borne avenues, maybe someone's developed this method without it being publicly known."

"Why have we never heard of this Kuru before?" asked Danny.

"There hasn't been much written on it, because it didn't impact us here in the US. Ever heard of Mad Cow disease?"

"Of course."

"Same thing, but when it threatened our way of life, everyone heard about it."

Sawyer stood up. "If what you're saying is true, and Ted down in the mailroom sneezed on someone—"

"Exactly," said Kira. "God, I hope I'm wrong."

"Wait," said Danny. "I do think you're wrong. Jacob told me his research showed no foreign infestations other than some ex-pats. I know the airline industry is struggling, but if it really was infectious, we would see a lot more of this in other countries."

"Might be too early. If it's got a latent period before symptoms occur, we might still see it spread. Can't be too careful. I'm going down to check out Ted," Sawyer said with as much bravado as he could feign.

He descended the stairs and walked through the mailroom door to see Amber with her back to him, sorting through mail with ear buds which made her unaware of his presence. As she bobbed her head in beat to unheard music, Sawyer found Ted's locker and opened it. His cell phone laid on the upper shelf. He glanced back at Amber, pocketed the phone, closed the locker door, and headed back upstairs.

29

Danny was surprised at the number of people on the streets. The weather app on his cell phone read a hundred and fifteen, and his steering wheel made from RIM pigmented urethane boasted a temperature within a few degrees of hell. He learned to carry gloves during the Arizona summers, choosing to sweat over playing hot potato while driving. Two fire trucks screamed past him as he turned onto south sixteenth street. About half of the ambulatory citizenry wore facemasks. Like Danny, they chose to sweat over increasing their odds of contracting the corona virus, now known as the delta variant.

He pulled up to the Central City Precinct where Mrs. Sandam was to be hanging out. He thought about calling her instead of locating her here, but knew her phone might be tapped, and even if it were not, he knew a face-to-face meeting would be best. As an ex-reporter, information gathering became easier when he was knee-to-knee, toe-to-toe with his interviewees.

He parked in the visitors' parking lot, perspired considerably on the way to the front door, showed his press credentials, and was escorted through the metal detector and into a Victorian-styled vacuous office with a faint aroma of lemon oil mixed with cigar smoke. "What can I do for you?" asked Commander John Lichtenfield. He sat behind an imposing desk which had been given to the precinct by The Very Reverend Connie Young when his congregation gave him a new marble desk for his twentieth anniversary. His neatly trimmed coal black hair was combed back to display an abnormally low hairline. His masseter muscles bulged from years of stressful clenching and his dark brown eyes appeared as if they could trespass into Danny's soul.

He chose to stand so as not to disappear from the commander's view. "I'm here to simply observe."

"Come now, Mr. King," he said with a husky voice a few octaves lower than Danny's, and a grin so fake Danny considered calling him on it. "Please be more specific."

"No, really. We're going to run a story in the Metro section on an average day at the precinct. I'm thinking of naming it," forming a large C with his right hand and sweeping it across his body, "Lichtenfield of Dreams: A City That Doesn't Sleep."

"Very clever, King." His grin quickly melted. "But perhaps in light of this insomnia flu, the double entendre might not be appreciated."

Danny shrugged. "I suppose you're right. Back to the drawing board on the headline, but my task hasn't changed. I'm still here to observe and I'll stay out of your hair."

"Just don't make a nuisance of yourself. Markovic! Show Mr. King out, and let the Sargent know he's free to observe, but no questions will be answered." He stared back at Danny and pierced his soul.

"Yes, sir," the stiffly postured officer said. Danny followed him out the door. Lichtenfield punched two buttons on his desk phone.

"Yes, John?"

"Sir, you wanted to know if anyone with the *Arizona Times Herald* showed up."

"What's going on?"

"Their executive editor, Danny King, says he's here to observe."

"That's fine. Just keep an eye on him and don't let him talk to the Sandam widow if she shows up."

Lichtenfield hesitated. "She's already here, and we don't know if she's a widow yet, sir."

"Sorry. Jumped to a damn conclusion. I just didn't see much hope of locating him alive at this point. Now get off this phone and see to it she and King don't talk. She's bat-shit crazy."

"Yes sir," Lichtenfield responded, but the connection was already severed. He walked out and down the hall toward the front desk. Seeing King and Sandam already talking, he yelled across the desk and over an officer on the phone who jumped at the outburst. "King! I've got something to show you. I think you'll appreciate it." The afternoon sun poured through the glass entry doors, and he squinted as he addressed the editor.

"I'll be right there," Danny said. He held his palm up. He had already slipped his card to Darcy Sandam and softened his voice as he spoke. "Don't come back here. Call me from your sister's cell phone—"

"How did you know I have a sister?"

"It's my job to know things. We'll meet at a site of your choosing. I may be able to help you." He glanced back at Lichtenfield and waved. "Gotta run, Commander! Forgot about a meeting!" He pivoted and strode out the door. He imagined the hostile look on his antagonist's face.

30

Livingston, Montana

A shirtless Bill Tumey sat in his living room with the television on the History channel, slacks laying at his feet, white boxers hiked up to his navel and a half-empty bottle of Jameson between his legs. Hashy, Enzo, and Henry were gone. His despair was a notch below his guilt, which was a notch below his fear. And his fear was electric. The whiskey designed to tamp down his emotions missed the mark. After a few more glasses, he transitioned into a hallucinatory phase, and began pleading for his gran-gran to make the see-saw stop. He soon forgot why he felt ruinous, just that he did. Whippoorwills sang to him through the window as the dusk of evening melted away to a dry and chilly night. The drone of the air conditioner lulled him to sleep, and as he collapsed onto the couch, his gran-gran sang him a lullaby. He did not move until the next morning after ten o'clock on July Fourth. It inched toward one hundred ten degrees, and he debated with himself. *Stay inside and get rid of this headache or*—his phone vibrated. When he saw who was calling, he let it buzz a few times, then reluctantly answered. "This is Bill."

"Thank you for your help, Mr. Tumey. We've given you a raise."

31

Phoenix, Arizona

Jacob rushed into his office as he saw his line blinking red through the window. *Forgot to shut the blinds again*, he mused to himself.

"This is Jacob."

"Is line secure?" asked a shaky voice with an Asian accent. He noticed a sticky note next to a cell phone which read:

> Ted left his phone in his locker. Think you should keep it so no one else gets access. Code is 1234. Sawyer

His mind returned to the question. *Sounds like a prank call, but I'll play this out.* "This isn't the government, so we can't afford that technology, but I have no reason to believe anyone's listening in." Jacob relaxed into his chair and pulled out his legal pad. He hoped there would be a reward for this effort.

"I feel much relief if you speak on phone removed from office. Use caller ID to call back from phone no connect to *Arizona Times Herald*." The connection ended, and Jacob made a note of the number. He turned on Ted's phone, charged it for a few minutes, then called the number back.

"Hello?"

"This is Jacob calling you back."

"Are you away from office?"

Jacob was tiring of the paranoia but decided to continue. "I'm on a secure phone but I'm in my private office."

"No repeat anything. Not name. I not know your office safe."

"Listen, just tell me something to get my attention and I'll decide if I need to worry about any more clandestine behavior."

After a pause, the voice said, "I know who responsible for insomnia flu in US and man who responsible for discovering how to transmit virus . . . someone kill him."

32

"Mr. King, a Darcy Sandam is on the phone. Should I take a message?"

"No! I'll take it, Jonie." Danny punched line two. "Thanks for calling Ms. Sandam. Is this your sister's phone?"

"Of course. I can follow instructions."

"I'm sorry. Just making sure. What can you tell me—"

"I'll only speak with Miss Quito present."

"Miss Quito?" Danny did not recognize the name.

"Jilian Quito. Senator Bonner's administrative assistant." She made the sign of the cross on the other end.

"I see. It's too risky to do a three-way call. Let me see when she can meet, and we'll work out a time and location. Are you generally free?"

"Yes, I spend most of my time at Central City, as you know, but I can't get anywhere with them, so you can happen on me there again, or take a chance on calling my phone. I'm not carrying my sister's around with me."

"Like I said, don't go back to the precinct," said Danny.

Darcy sobbed softly. "Mr. King, this isn't my kind of thing, but now you're scaring me."

"It's okay. Maybe I've read too many spy novels, but you can't be too careful. I'm sure there's no danger, so hang tight and I'll text you the time and location."

"There's a dry cleaner. Shanghai. It shut down after COVID hit. It's on the corner of Bell and Jade. I know the owner and he can leave it unlocked for us."

"Sounds good. I'll text you a time once I work it out with Jilian."

"I trust you, Mr. King."

Danny ended the call, then stood and walked to Jacob's office, seeing he was just hanging up his phone. He stood in front of his door until Jacob waved him in. "You busy?"

"I'm sorry." Jacob's mind was elsewhere. "What was that?"

"I just asked if you were busy, but I see you're a bit pre-occupied."

"Sorry. Just got a call from someone who claims he knows how the virus started and knows the guy who discovered the method for transmission." He shook his head slowly.

"Why aren't you more excited? This is great news!"

Jacob sighed. "The guy's dead."

"Good god. Can this get any more strange?"

"I hear ya. But what have you got?"

Danny closed the door behind him and pulled a chair from the corner to the front of Jacob's desk and sat. "Do you know a Miss Jilian Quito with the senator's office?"

"Yes, I do."

"Well, I've been in contact with the Sandam widow and she's willing to talk to me, but only with Jilian."

"I see." Jacob's attention disappeared as he gazed out his window. A few seconds later, he continued. "By all means, set up a meeting."

Danny was puzzled by his matter-of-fact response and lack of inquisitiveness. "I can see you have a lot to work through. I'll get out of your hair if you'll get me Jilian's contact info."

"It's in the google doc file called 'insomnia flu'. Let me know if you can't locate it."

"Thanks, Jacob." Danny rose. "Sounds like we might have a breakthrough with that call. Let me know if you need any help."

Jacob stared out the window again. "I'm sorry, Danny. What was that?"

"Never mind." Danny waved his hand and headed through the door. "Just let me know if you need anything!"

33

Scottsdale, Arizona

The two men sat on either side of a white marble table in a palatial estate on Cintarosa Pass. A conference phone sat between them, inanimate, but it held the attention of both men as they awaited the call. The chef, the maids, and even the security detail had been given the day off.

The phone buzzed and the one with the thinning white hair punched the flashing red button. "Is that you, Antioch?"

There was a pause before a gravelly voice responded. "Status!" was the extent of his reply.

"No worries," said the one wearing a beige jumpsuit. "You know the phone is secure. My man checked for bugs before he left and it's just us three here. House is locked down tight."

"Good. Falcon, what's the latest on—"

"Let me stop you right there," said the white-headed man known as Falcon. "I've got an agenda here I think will answer most questions. Let me work through this chronologically and if there's anything I've left out, you can ask when I'm done."

"Let's get this moving. I've got a flight in two hours."

"Shouldn't be a problem. Number one, we've scrubbed the internet of anything that could tie us to ZPG. There wasn't much, but it's cleaner than my girlfriend's—"

"Don't need to know that, Falcon."

"Number two. Genesis has been eliminated. Number—"

"Did we use the Salamander?"

"Of course. He arrived from Milan last week and will be available until the 23rd. Three. Judge Stoutmeyer will not be filling the Senator's seat. I've appointed Bradley. Number—"

"Wait. Need more information on that. It would appear we have some loose ends."

"Astute observation, Antioch." Falcon glanced at the one in the jumpsuit. "You might appreciate the breadth of the senator's tentacles was impressive, and, unfortunately, not transparent. It would be impossible to blind everyone, but we've purposely created loose ends where necessary. We have someone on the inside who'll be alerting us to any hint of discovery."

Antioch's voice raised, making his gravelly tenor sound painful. "Do I need to remind you what could happen if either of you turn state's evidence?"

They both hesitated while deciding how to respond. "Of course," said the jumpsuited one as he ran his hand through coiffed gray hair. "We have no interest in implicating anyone . . . and yes, we know what you can do."

"What else is on your agenda?"

"Realized revenue from the site as of this morning is a tic over 47 million."

"Projected X by next month?"

Falcon beamed. "We're looking at seven X, and the next month should be fourteen X. That puts us at 4.5 billion by September."

"Any investigatory concerns?"

Poseidon glanced at Falcon, then responded. "Not yet, Antioch, but once it crosses one hundred million, we expect some inquiries, just like we discussed."

"Good to hear. We have contingencies for that, but I'd rather hold off for now."

"We agree," said Falcon. "Last item is a decision on what to do with thirty-seven. Poseidon thinks we can still use him."

The gray-haired man quickly inserted, "Yes, he has some connections he could help us with and—"

"I don't give a fuck about connections. Thirty-seven is just another number in need of disappearing. Is that clear?"

"It is," said Poseidon quickly.

"If that's all, I'm headed to the airport. Don't contact me again unless something gets fucked up. No, forget that. Just fix it if it does. Only contact me with good news." The connection ended.

"About what I expected," Falcon said. "I'll take care of thirty-seven."

34

Phoenix, Arizona

It was another sweltering day which choked the energy and will out of even the best of intentions. Danny wondered how mankind functioned in this area of the world before circulating air was invented, but he did not dwell on this for long, as Darcy Sandam entered the Shanghai Dry Cleaners a few seconds after him. She stood six inches taller than Danny. "Good afternoon, Ms. Sandam. I know what you're thinking, and Ms. Quito will be here shortly." She nodded and said nothing. "Would you like to go back to the room or—"

"I'll wait for her here," she said.

"Of course. Have any trouble getting here?" He knew Darcy's trust in him was volatile. The effects of stress on her health were obvious. Deep circles underscored sad, hazel-colored eyes. She displayed a slumped countenance which betrayed her once-defiant persona. Her words exited painfully.

"Not at all. I used to bring Kevin's suits here—"

"Sorry, Darcy. Didn't mean to dredge up uncomfortable memories."

"No, no. That's fine. I stopped bringing anything in when Kevin stopped traveling for work. The owner here is a friend. Faustino is his name. Told me he held on as long as he could, but when everyone stopped traveling during the pandemic, no one needed their suits cleaned, so he was forced to close a business he owned for twenty—"

The door swung open, and Jilian walked in. "Glad they left the AC on in here. You must be Danny with the *Arizona Times Herald*." They shook hands.

"Let's go back to the office," Danny said as he walked ahead of the ladies. Jilian hugged Darcy before they found seats.

"How are you holding up?" Jilian put a hand on Darcy's left arm.

"Not well. Can't sleep at all." Danny regarded her with concern. "No, it's not the virus, Mr. King. It's depression and anxiety. Are you married, Mr. King?"

"Only married to my job now, Ms. Sandam," Danny said with a hint of remorse.

"I see. Kevin's been missing for seventeen days now. As cold as this may sound, I'd sleep better if I knew he was dead. It's the *not* knowing that won't allow me any closure. It's tying me in knots."

"If I may say," Jilian began, "before the senator got sick, since she knew Governor Adair's budget director, she called in a favor and got Kevin on his staff. He became a favored son of the director, and when the director announced his retirement four months ago, he pushed for Kevin to take his place. Just before he was to take over, he disappeared. Sadly, I never got to meet Kevin."

"Anything to add or subtract from that, Ms. Sandam?" Danny asked.

"Only that he called me on that Tuesday from his office and sounded upset." She pulled a photo out of her billfold of she and Kevin which was taken a few years ago at a beach bar and handed it to Danny. "He didn't say anything disturbing, but I've known him for nine years. I know he's saying something without saying it. I wish he had because I haven't seen him since. He never made it home that night." She wiped away some tears which leaked from her swollen eyelids.

It was Danny's turn to place a hand on Darcy's arm. "We're here to help you, Ms. Sandam. We're investigating the police depart—"

"Fuck the police!" Darcy cried.

"I understand how you feel," Danny said. "We're also investigating the governor. My guess is your husband was getting too close."

Darcy Sandam turned to Jilian. "What did Senator Bonner ask of my husband?"

This caught her off guard. "Well . . . she didn't tell me everything, but—"

"Don't hide behind that veil, Ms. Quito. I'm quite sure she provided plenty of details. You were her communications director. I beg you. Please don't hide anything from me."

Jilian paused before continuing. "I'm sorry. I only meant I have no way of knowing if she kept anything from me. What I *do* know is she uncovered an entity known as the Klavian Triumvirate. They were, or I suppose still are, a secret group—a set of three puppet masters pulling some dangerous strings."

"And that's who we're focusing on, Ms. Sandam," Danny said. "I have my best—"

His words were choked off as an explosion ripped through the office wall. It projected clothing-rack metal and drywall at a rate of speed leaving no time for reaction. The three were trajected into the opposing wall before the ceiling and second floor collapsed. As the dust settled, sirens in the distance wailed an ominous testimony that all was not well.

35

He punched the blinking red button. "Jacob."

"Sir, this is the Phoenix Fire Department. We've been told by a Miss Jilian Quito to call you about Danny King."

"Oh my god. What happened?" Jacob tensed as he heard sirens and commotion on the other end of the line.

"There was an explosion in a dry cleaner store on Bell Road. Mr. King is severely injured, and he's been e-vacced to Banner University. He was unconscious when I saw him leave on a stretcher."

Jacob stared at the phone and willed the voice to go away. *This can't be happening.*

"Mr. Potter?"

"How is Miss Quito?"

"We have one deceased female. Miss Quito has a fractured arm and broken ribs along with many lacerations, but she will live. She told us the name of the deceased, but I can't release that information until the next of kin has been notified."

"Where are you taking Miss Quito?"

"Same hospital. It's the closest."

"Headed there." Jacob ended the connection, picked up his keys and took the elevator down to the parking garage. His mind raced as he tried to connect the dots between Sylvia and now Danny. Taking his mind off the confusion playing out before him, he used voice commands to text Wendy.

> Headed to hospital. Danny's been injured. Let you know when I know more.

To keep from spiraling into negativity, he would often mentally retreat to his uncle Sidney's ranch. He revisited a time when he had a goal one morning to break his record of feral hog kills. After locating the den, he found a good prop for his rifle in the fork of a juniper tree and waited. Soon, a hog exited and was put down with one expert shot to the neck. When the next one came out soon after, he aimed and pulled the trigger, but it didn't fire. He released the shell and inserted another, but the gun refused to fire. It was at this time that he realized he was upwind from the den—a mistake he quickly understood realized would create a tense chain of events.

More hogs exited, holding their snouts in the air and sniffing. They sensed danger with a fallen friend and the smell of blood close by. Smelling the smoke from the first shot, they trotted toward young Jacob. He tried a third shell with no luck.

The memory faded as he parked near the emergency wing and hurried through the door. He found the first person in scrubs and asked, "Was Danny King brought in?"

"We've had several come through here. Are you related to this Mr. King?"

"Yes. He's my little brother," Jacob lied.

"Talk to the registrar over there." She pointed to a closed plexiglass window with no one behind it. Jacob rushed over and peered through, then rapped on the window several times. A man in uniform approached the window and said through the closed plexiglass, "Sir, you'll have to be patient. Someone will be here shortly." He turned and left Jacob standing.

Calm down, Jacob. Use the Optavia maneuver.

He waited for the next hospital employee to walk through the door. He did not have to wait long. A man with a Givenchy suit, red tie, and Banner Hospital nametag walked out, and Jacob caught him by surprise. "Do you know who the PR person is here at the hospital? I'm with the *Arizona Times Herald*," holding out his creds, "and we're doing a piece on why this hospital was ranked number one in the most recent oleander national poll. This hospital is the pride of Arizona. Who can I speak with to get some quotes and material for the Sunday edition?"

"Mr. . . . Potter. This is hardly the place to locate the one you seek. I suggest—"

"Mr. Reynolds. Yes, this might strike you as an odd request under the circumstances, but I just came to see one of my employees who was admitted, and—"

"Did you get to see them?"

"No, since I'm not family."

"Come with me." He turned and walked back through the door. Jacob slid through behind him. Reynolds glanced back over his shoulder and asked, "Name of your employee?"

"King. Danny King."

"Wait here." Jacob stood at a counter behind which personnel were busy at their computers. An oversized atomic clock was high enough on a wall for all to see it. He hated clocks. His disdain, though idiosyncratic, was severe. Hated them with such passion that no clocks were allowed in the *Arizona Times Herald* offices. In a few minutes, a physician walked through the double doors and angled toward him.

"Mr. Potter?"

"Yes?" Jacob straightened.

"This is not standard procedure, but we have been unable to contact any of Mr. King's next of kin."

"What happened?"

"Please, Mr. Potter, what we need is your help in locating anyone related—"

"He has no relatives!" Jacob cut him off. "His parents are dead, he was an only child; no children, and his wife left him, and disappeared. Now will you please tell me how he's doing?"

The doctor avoided Jacob's eyes. "He didn't make it, Mr. Potter. I'm so sorry." He slowly turned and walked back through the doors. He offered no more words of explanation or condolence.

Jacob sat in a chair and covered his face with his hands. He shut out the patter from the computers and the hum of the central air which worked overtime in triple digit Arizona. His mind raced between incongruous thoughts. *What if something like this happened to Wendy? Did Danny suffer? Dying without any family is awful. What would it feel like to be crushed inside a collapsed building? Did Reynolds leave? Would Danny's wife even care? Should I try to find her? This doesn't make any sense. Quito will be in surgery . . . have to get to her before the police do.*

He thought about his uncle Sidney. He had been a man of prayer, and when the *Arizona Times Herald*, the family, or the baseball team found itself in need of a heartfelt plea, Sidney responded. His words flowed effortlessly, like a mountain stream flows over rocks without slowing or faltering. *Wish I could pray like Uncle Sidney now.* Instead, he rose and walked out of the hospital.

36

Bill stepped out of the RV he had rented from Hunderlee's Movables on Tuesday, paid cash, and used the name Gary Snively. He parked in an abandoned campsite, in the shadows of Camelback Mountain, then wondered if he would ever feel safe again. A crack of thunder made him twitch. *This is crazy. I can't live like this.* He had the eight hundred thousand which was deposited into his account the day before, but how long would that last?

Returning to *The Joint Joint* was out of the question, so that twenty-year investment would soon become insolvent. He felt a tinge of guilt for leaving employees without a job, but he easily rationalized. Delores only worked for him so she could partake of his inventory. Judy was a busybody who was always late and had a laugh which set his nerves on edge. Besides, she was always hinting she wanted to move back to Palm Beach. He could leave Arizona, but would they track him down? He could go to authorities, but without proof and without names . . . He decided to stay for a few days. No one knew he was here, and he had enough food and water to last a few weeks.

What have I done?

37

Jacob entered the *Arizona Times Herald* floor and saw the news of Danny's death preceded him. Danny would often shoot before he aimed, which left people guessing and often doubting. Jacob often said to the team that Danny King was their boss, but they were tasked with keeping "the King" in check. Jacob's love of chess often bled over to the newspaper business.

Sylvia . . . and now Danny. One dead because of InF and one because he was investigating it? This is insane. Whoever they are, I'm not letting them beat me.

Without saying a word, he hustled down the stairs to the mailroom, found Ted's locker and located his phone. He was relieved to see his sister had not come up to claim it. He turned it on, using 1234 as the password and found the text he was searching for.

Flying to U.S. on Wednesday. Meet at Marriott rm 346 at 7PM. Come alone. Friend of Enzo

He typed,

See you at 7 Wednesday. Jacob Potter.

He decided to keep the phone for the time being and stuffed it into his pocket. He headed back up the stairs, meeting Kira who was headed down. "Mr. Potter, I'm so sorry to hear about Danny. What would you like Sawyer and me to do now?"

Jacob stood in the stairwell with her and decided that was as good as anyplace to have a sensitive discussion. "Not sure where you are with your current assignment, but right now, I need you to head to Banner and wait for Jilian Quito to come out of surgery. Call me the minute she comes out and I'll head there. We have to talk to her before the police do."

"Yes sir. I should be there in fifteen minutes." She turned and hurried up the stairs.

He stood without moving in the stairwell for a few minutes and enjoyed the solitude. He did not want to go up and field a constellation of questions for which he had no answers. He worried about others, Kira and Sawyer especially. *Am I endangering others by not going to the police? Was the explosion just an accident? If not, who was it meant for?* When he did make it back to his desk, he realized his concerns were not to materialize. No one wanted to discuss Danny's death. Perhaps it was the lack of respect for someone who, when alive, did little to earn it. Perhaps their grieving quotient for the week was used up on Sylvia. Whatever the reasons, he was relieved.

He spent a few hours mapping out the next few days' itinerary for the *Arizona Times Herald* and, without a clock in sight, headed home for a potent alcoholic beverage, playing the gait song, "It's Five O'Clock Somewhere," as he walked up his sidewalk. Wendy was at her weekly bunco party and would not be home until late. She never approved of his beeline to the bourbon selection when arriving home after a trying day, so he warmly anticipated the absence of her sideways glance. A closet introvert, he lusted after parcels of time where he could regain his energy through solitude. He made himself an old-fashioned and turned on ESPN as he propped up his feet on the ottoman—something he was not allowed to do when Wendy was home. With bourbon flowing through his veins, the memories of the day faded to a blur and allowed him to separate himself from the job and enjoy his Phoenix Suns playing the Dallas Mavericks. The fact his team was losing by twenty at the half mattered not. At 8:35 p.m., his alone time was interrupted by the doorbell. *Never good when someone stops by this late.*

He turned off the television and opened the door to observe Marie sitting on a statue of a lion in the front lawn which Jacob had received from the Lions Club.

"Came by for a drinkie-poo," she slurred. "What have you got?"

"Sounds like we need to talk," he said as he placed her arm over his shoulder, his hand around her waist, and helped her inside. *I hope no one's taking photos.* He successfully situated her in a sofa chair by the fireplace, then said reproachfully, "Marie. What's this all about?"

"Do you have any vodka? That makes me drink more clearly . . . think . . . more . . . where was I?"

"Let's talk first. When I discover why you're here in this inebriated state, I'll see what I can do."

Marie's face turned into an exaggerated pout. "You don't have to be so mean."

"Are you even capable of telling me what this is all about? And how did you know where I live?"

She weaved on the chair before responding. "Like you said, I'd make a great newspepper personage. I know things. Know something else I know?"

"What's that, Marie?"

"I forgot . . . oh, I remember just now. I know I need to throw up."

Jacob quickly ushered her to the bathroom, lifted the lid on the toilet, and positioned her on her knees. She placed her hands on the side of the bowl and relieved her stomach of the quinoa salad and hummus she had for dinner. Jacob handed her a wet rag and they returned to the living room.

"Now can you tell me what's going on?"

Marie leaned her head back in the chair and wiped moisture from her eyes. She struggled to speak, less a function of the alcohol than the pain she was in. "My older sister passed away last night."

"I'm so sorry, Marie."

"No one even told me she was shick. She lives in Newwww . . . Hampshire and we both have busy busy busy lives. We don't talk too often. Pretty sure she had that skanky insomnia flu."

"How long was she sick?"

"My m . . . mother said maybe threety months, but she . . . really didn't know either. Jacob. Nail these bastards!"

Jacob considered telling her about Danny but thought better of it. "You're sure this isn't hereditary or infectious? On second thought, I shouldn't be asking you questions with you in this state. I need to get you home."

"I have my car," Marie said as she attempted to rise from the chair.

"You're not driving home. You can get your car tomorrow." He led her to his Subaru in the garage and asked if she could remember her address.

"Don't be silly. It's . . . let me check my phone." She found her address and clumsily handed the phone to Jacob. "I'm s. . . . sorry about your toilet, Potters."

After he deposited her inside the front door, trusting she could handle locating her own bed, he headed home to answer questions from Wendy about a strange car parked on their front lawn. It was not the easiest or least argumentative discourse of their twelve-year marriage.

38

The next morning, at 7:25, Jacob called Kira. "Was Jilian in surgery all night?"

"No, but they weren't allowing anyone to see her. I slept off and on in the reception area, but just checked again and got stonewalled."

"I'm on my way!" Jacob ended the call, dressed quickly, put some clothes in a bag and began the twenty-minute drive to Banner University Hospital. He thought about calling Marie, but as this was Saturday, he estimated her hangover headache would keep her down till noon. He was surprised to see her name appear as his cell played *Doctor Doctor* by Robert Palmer. He felt lucky Wendy, even if she had been in the car, was unfamiliar with the lyrics.

"How's your head this morning, Marie?"

"Fine. Rode my bike twenty-five miles before the sun came up. Helped to clear my head. I'm calling to see how I can help. Cleared the rest of the day."

Jacob reminisced of decades earlier when he could lay one on and get back in the saddle the next morning. "Do you have privileges at Banner?"

"Only courtesy, but I've been able to visit my InF patients there with no problem."

"If you want to help, meet me at Banner as soon as you can. Bring your doctor jacket or whatever you call that thing."

"I just stepped out of the shower. Be there in thirty. Tops."

Ten minutes later, she called again. "Didn't want to waste time earlier, but can you fill me in now?"

Jacob spent the last five minutes of his trip presenting what little he knew of the Klavian Triumvirate, the explosion, and Kevin Sandam's disappearance. "Marie, I'm here now. I'll try to lay some groundwork before you get here."

Kira was waiting for him on the fourth floor at the nurse's station. "She's in room 418." She pointed down a hall which, in addition to some sparse traffic, revealed a suited man with arms folded sitting in a chair in front of one of the rooms. The seams of his navy sport coat were stressed to the limit by shoulders and arms begging for escape.

"Who's our bouncer?"

"Not sure, but he's not FBI nor police. No gun, no badge, and he refuses to show any ID. Just said he's got strict orders. Says only medical personnel allowed inside."

Jacob smiled mischievously. "Got that taken care of. He turned to the nurse behind the desk, and said, "Nurse . . . Oliphant?"

"Yes, how can I help you?" She had a pleasant smile.

"Dr. Marie Jimmerson is my sister's internist. Have you seen her?"

The nurse raised her eyebrows. "I don't know a Dr. Jimmerson, and who is your sister?"

"I'm sorry. My sister is Jilian Quito, and—"

"Ms. Quito is to be left undisturbed."

"I understand, but the doctor who is treating her insomnia flu is on her way. She wanted me to meet her here as next of kin.

I'm afraid she doesn't have long to live." Jacob's efforts to appear sincere were successful.

"I'm so sorry. I didn't realize she contracted the insomnia flu. It's a good thing she's in a private room."

They turned as Marie walked up behind them. Her ankle-length clinic jacket was buttoned, her hair pulled back into a bun, and she had grabbed a clipboard from her back seat which held little of her attention. "I don't have much time. I have a reception area full of InF patients back at the office, but none as far along the spectrum as your sister, Mr. Potter. I'll do my best to make her comfortable." She turned to nurse Oliphant. "Can you please tell me what room Ms. Quito is in?"

The nurse hesitated, then rose and uneasily walked through a swinging door and motioned Marie to follow her. When Jacob and Kira started to follow as well, she turned and started to object, but stopped and continued to the room. Jacob mentally turned on "Stayin' Alive" by the Bee Gees for his gait song. As she approached room 418, the sitting guard rose, and Jacob was surprised to see he stood a good six inches taller than his six-foot four frame. Jacob played four years of basketball at Albany State, averaging twenty-six points his senior year, but as it was a division two school, he went unnoticed by NBA scouts. He moved to Phoenix to carry on his uncle's newspaper business, but in his years at Albany, he rarely struggled to navigate around the taller, less agile players on his way to the rim. He hoped this guy would pose equally minimal deterrence.

"Who are these people, nurse?"

"This is Dr—"

"Jimmerson," Marie said.

"Sorry. Dr. Jimmerson is Ms. Quito's internist. She's here to check on the condition of her insomnia flu."

The tall man swiped a blond bang out of his left eye and regarded each person standing. "No one told me she had that flu."

"Did anyone ask her?" Marie asked.

"I'm not her doctor, so—"

"Well, I am. Please let us in, sir. She may not make it through the night, and I would like her brother and niece to come with me. We won't be long."

He glanced down the hall, then to nurse Oliphant who shrugged her shoulders. "All right, Dr. Jimmerson. I'll give you five minutes."

Marie charged through the door before he finished and without acknowledging him. Jacob and Kira followed and allowed the door to swing closed. Jacob hurried to the bathroom, removed the toilet roll from the holder and stuffed it into the commode, sliding it back until it wedged. He dried his hands with paper towels and closed the door, then walked to the white clock on the wall and turned it around.

His audience followed his moves. "What was that all about?" asked Jilian.

"He hates clocks," Kira said.

"But the toilet?"

In a hushed voice, Jacob ignored the question. "We don't have much time, but this is Kira from the *Arizona Times Herald*, and this is Marie Jimmerson. She's a real doc, by the way. Kira's been here all day, and all signs say we'll have to get you out of here. That explosion was no accident, and we don't want someone to come back here and finish the job. They think you have the insomnia flu, so that could buy us some time, but you have to play sick. Can you walk?"

"My arm took all the punishment," Jilian said. "I should be fine. By the way, Darcy had a photo of her and Kevin in the dry cleaners. The staff here must have thought it was mine because it was left on my cart when I woke up. Do you need it for any reason?"

Jacob took the photo and inspected it. Marie peered over his shoulder at the two in the photo who posed awkwardly, resembling more closely a brother and sister at odds instead of a happily married couple. "I'll take it, Jilian."

"So, what's the plan?" she asked.

"In a minute, Kira is going to exit and walk to the restroom by the elevators." He turned to Kira. "Make sure no one sees you go in and take this bag with you." She nodded.

"Just before we leave, I'm going to go to the restroom in here. Don't let this gross you out, but I've been holding it in and when I flush and leave, it's going to get ugly in here real quick." Kira slapped her hand over her mouth to keep from audibly gagging. "You'll be fine, Kira. It's Jilian we need to worry about. Jilian, after we leave and the floor floods, call the nurse's station and sound desperate."

"That won't be difficult."

"That's what I'm counting on. Tell them your room is flooded and you must use the restroom right now. You don't have a catheter, do you?"

"No, they took it out this morning."

"Good. I was counting on that. Have you had any conversations with the gentleman in front of your door? Or Nurse Oliphant?"

"I doubt it. The nurses changed over this morning, and no one's been in. I didn't even know there was a guy in front of my room."

"Perfect. The nurse should take you to the same restroom by the elevator. If not, just tell her you left your brush in that one last night and need to retrieve it. Kira, I asked you to be here because you and Jilian are about the same size." He moved his eyes between them. "And your hair color is close."

"Uh-oh. I see where this is going." Kira shook her head.

"Yep. I need you and Jilian to switch clothes, sling and all. The masks will do the rest, but I have a surgical cap here for insurance. Put it on now, Jilian. You'll give it to Kira in the restroom. We leave by the elevators as soon as Kira is headed back to the room. Everyone clear?"

Kira responded. "You gonna address the elephant in the room?"

"You mean what happens to you when they discover you aren't Jilian?"

"Yeah. Will they cart me off to jail?"

"No. There is no police presence and I have a plan for getting you back sooner anyway." He reached into the bag he handed Kira and lifted the contents. "These should fit. It's a skirt, blouse, and loose moccasins. They can't bring you back to this room until they get it cleaned up. Ask if you can sit in the waiting room while it gets cleaned. Before you leave the restroom by the elevator, put the clothes under your gown. When you've been sitting in the waiting room for a few minutes—I'm sure you'll have our guy outside as an escort—just hoping he doesn't follow you into the bathroom in that area. Tell him the orange juice they gave you for breakfast must have been a diuretic. Don't be shocked if that doesn't compute with him. When you're in the stall, change into the skirt and blouse, remove the sling and surgical cap, then dump it all in the trash can before walking out. Don't acknowledge the idiot. Get in your car, and . . ." He swiveled to Marie. "Can we take Jilian to your house?"

"Might not be best. Since I'm here, they might try to track me down. I suggest we take her to a friend of mine, Dr. Kyle Hunter. He can also attend to Jilian's injuries."

"Can we trust him?" Jacob asked.

"Yes. We've been talking about the insomnia flu and the potential cover up. He rode with me this morning on our bike ride."

"Great. Text me his address and meet us there. We'll wait
outside until you arrive. Everyone ready?" They all nodded. "Good
luck, Kira." She confidently walked out the door.

The plan worked almost without incident. When brown
water ran under the door to the hall, Kira didn't have to make the
call. Pandemonium ensued as traffic along the hall was effectively
unnavigable. Personnel brought Kira a respirator mask until they
were able to clear and sanitize the room. The plumber was flum-
moxed, as after Jacob had flushed seven times, then bolted, the
toilet roll softened and worked loose, then spilled over and floated
into a corner. They attempted to place Kira in a new room, but
she made a scene, arguing she had arranged everything feng shui
and 418 was meant to be her room because her mother's birthday
was on April 18th. She simply had to have room 418. This gave
her some time in the waiting room, where she edited the plan and
asked to use the restroom when they arrived instead of after a few
minutes. She reasoned correctly if her escort did not see anyone
else enter the restroom, he might be suspicious. As it was, she only
received a sideways glance from the guard as she exited.

39

They met at Kyle's house at 4:35, shortly before he drove up after leaving the office early. A treehouse had been built, which cantilevered over his long driveway. Visitors nervously drove under it quickly as they imagined it collapsing on que. Once acquaintances were made inside, Kyle gave Jilian a sling he brought from his office and changed a few bandages.

"Pizza good with everyone? I've got an oven in my outdoor kitchen, and they taste better than anything we could get on short notice. Can't explain why the pizza tastes better when it's cooked outside. Just have to trust me."

All agreed that sounded good.

As he prepared two large deep-dish concoctions he called Hunter Surprises in the kitchen, Jilian said, "I have more information from the senator. I only held back because I didn't know who to trust, but my thoughts on that have changed."

They were seated around a replica of the Dunder Mifflin conference room table. No one knew of Dr. Hunter's obsession with *The Office* nor the significance of the oval piece of furniture, but that mattered little to Kyle.

"Mind if I take notes?" Jacob asked.

"As long as you don't record or quote me," said Quito.

"You have my word."

She rearranged herself in the chair. "Let's start with Kevin Sandam. His wife was killed in the explosion I was in. Now that Darcy is no longer with us, I can tell you Kevin was having an affair with Governor Adair's chief of staff." This kicked the intensity level of the atmosphere up a notch.

"You mean Albert Leto?"

"Yes. He told Senator Bonner he developed the relationship to get more information on the governor, but the senator was never sold on this, and by the way, the information I'm sharing is all from the note she left for me to read after her death."

"Do you know why she didn't share this with you before her death?" Kira asked.

"She told me in the note she was only trying to protect me. Some of this information is so sensitive that it could cost me once I've shared it. The senator gave me permission not to, if only to save me from harm, but I thought it was too important to bury."

Jilian Quito was the fourth child born into a military family stationed in Okinawa. Both of her parents were also children of Marine parents, and when she became the first girl in three generations, much was expected. Since she was only one pound, eight ounces at birth, the family knew if she could win the fight to stay alive, she would conquer the world. Expectations were always high, and her trajectory was tenable, so she carried a healthy amount of anxiety into escalated affairs.

"Don't feel like you have to share," said Jacob. "But we will be most discreet with anything you tell us."

"Thank you, Mr. Potter. I appreciate—"

"Can we ask questions, Miss Quito?" Kyle asked as he returned from putting the pizzas in the oven.

"Of course."

"Maybe you've told the others, but how did someone come to place a bomb in that laundry where you had a meeting? Who knew about this, because from what I've learned, it was planted before you three arrived, and it was detonated remotely?"

"You appear to be quite knowledgeable about this, Dr. Hunter."

"My son-in-law works at the Cactus Park precinct, so I called him when I heard about the explosion. You were very fortunate."

"I do feel God's got something here for me. Wasn't my time. I think I'm to carry on the work of Senator Bonner. Oh, and by the way, it was Darcy's suggestion for where to meet. Maybe her contacts need to be investigated."

"What else was in the senator's note?" Jacob asked.

From the way each of them pivoted in her direction, it became clear all were equally curious.

Jilian smiled. "Another item about Kevin Sandam. He was asked by the governor's office to remove all references to a splinter faction of the Zero Population Group from the internet. Apparently, Kevin had a background in cybersecurity—some company named Idemica—it helped elevate his position more than anything. Spent a few years in Iraq, too. The package apparently impressed the governor. I'm not sure where it went sideways, but from what Darcy told me, he was acting like a different person for about a week before he disappeared."

Jacob appeared confused as his eyebrows wrinkled. "Sandam told you he was asked to erase evidence of the splinter group? Why didn't she—"

"I'm sorry. No, Darcy told me that part. It was odd, actually. She mentioned it when she referred to that week he wasn't himself.

She heard him talking to someone on his cell about it, and all she could tell was that he was agreeing to something. When he was in the shower the next day, she listened to the phone call. She never asked him about it, but she did say the call seemed strange. There was no mention of the other guy's name. It was to the point. Nothing else was discussed."

"Doesn't sound that unusual to me," said Marie. "But how the heck do you listen to a call that wasn't a voice mail?"

"I asked her that also. She used to work for AT&T in management and she called in a favor. She did say that she had to call from one of the phones that were used, though. I think it was a CYA thing with the AT&T friend."

"Did you get a name of that friend?" asked Jacob.

"No, I'm afraid not."

"Anything else on Sandam?"

"That's all Senator Bonner shared with me. I'm sure she knew little else."

Jacob reviewed his notes. "How did the senator discover Kevin Sandam to begin with?"

"Great question. Unfortunately, I can't be of much help. She mentioned his name one day about a year ago. . . even before she got sick. Said he had been referred to her as a potential head of her cybersecurity detail. She needed to vet him thoroughly before considering him. I helped her, but we went in another direction. He turned up clean, but she went with Nate Beard. She did use him with some contract work, but it was sporadic. I'm not sure why she pulled him in to try and get close to Governor Adair. As I said before, I think she was only trying to protect me, especially as her sickness became evident."

"Thank you, Ms. Quito. I appreciate—"

"You're leaving my name out of this, right?"

"Of course," Jacob reassured her. "I may say *anonymous source* but may not. Usually sounds like lazy reporting." He wrote down a few more notes, then regarded Marie. "I'm told your sister passed away yesterday." He carefully avoided any discussion of her inebriated visit to his home the night before. "Will you be flying to New York for the funeral?"

"No," Marie said. "The family's being paranoid. With COVID and now the insomnia flu, they're all hunkered down. Not even leaving the house. They're having the funeral home cremate her and keep the urn until they feel comfortable going to pick it up."

"I'm sorry to hear about your sister, Marie," Kyle offered. "I didn't even know you *had* a sister. Were you close?"

"Not really. Long story I don't need to rehash right now."

The story was not long but sharing it could lead to another embarrassing evening laced with alcohol, so she stiff-armed his question. She called Marsha Jimmerson her older sister, but she was only older by seventeen minutes. The disparate careers of the twin sisters created a festering and irreversible rift between them.

Over the years since their graduation from Southeast High in Bradenton, Florida, Marie's hunger for learning and a commitment to health contrasted arrantly with Marsha's desire to party and eschew college. Marsha showed passive-aggressive behavior by posting pictures of her three-hundred-pound body and claiming her twin was "even fatter." Their parents gave up trying to help Marsha over time, and Marie never lost the guilt over being the favored daughter. With a mother who wore size eighteen dresses, Marie knew genetics were not her friend. To Kyle, her cycling partner, she confided she would always be "riding away from the fat girl."

"Dr. Hunter," Jacob said. "I hate to impose, but could you put up Jilian and Marie here tonight? We're worried for their safety."

"Of course. With our two daughters gone, we have plenty of room. They can stay as long as they like. If you guys like to fish, my lake behind the house supports plenty of bass and catfish."

"Thank you," said Jilian. "We won't overstay our welcome, but maybe a few days until we know the difference between smoke and fire will help."

40

As the shadow of Camelback Mountain crawled over Bill's camper, he decided to begin his journey to West Virginia. Sitting and waiting created a level of anxiety he had never experienced. He always considered himself emotionally solid with no baggage to lay at the feet of a sympathetic therapist. Now? His mind turned grasshopper chirping to machine gunfire and the stars to incoming missiles.

He had taken a prophylactic nap during his 1:45 to 3:45 sleep gate in preparation for his all-night drive. He was marginally concerned anyone knew of his location or intentions, but he took no chances. His benefactors had killed with little hesitation, so he knew they would not think twice about eliminating someone who was a potential thorn. Bill had never given them reason to be placed in that position, but he knew they needed no reason.

He pulled out onto Camelback Road as the cooled breeze sliding off the mountain eased through his windows and delivered a message. He was not alone. He shivered, then sped down Highway 101 with the windows rolled up.

41

"I've got some data from the Rutherford Group, Jacob." Sawyer entered his office the next morning with Kira. They had spent the last twelve hours properly grieving Danny in their own way. They could have done it in twenty minutes.

"What have you got?"

"The most important numbers they gave me. There's a 98.7 percent predictive value the InF pandemic—and yes, they called it a pandemic—is intentional. It couldn't have happened by accident. Or at least it's extremely unlikely."

"Anything else?" This news did not come as a surprise to Jacob.

"The only other interesting data point was seventy-two percent of InF deaths have been female. It's the only outlier they found which had no reasonable explanation."

Jacob thought it best not to mention the previous day's activities to Sawyer. It became obvious to him Kira had not offered either. Marie and Jilian checked in from Kyle's place and reported no excitement. He was slated to meet with Luca today, another event he thought best concealed as his internal antennas were on full alert. He rifled through some papers on his desk, then said, "You'll have to excuse me now, but I've got some work to do and a meeting to prepare for."

"We'll get out of your hair," Sawyer said. They both turned and walked back through the door.

Jacob picked up his phone and texted Luca.

Meeting still on?

Yes

Room 346 at Marriott? 3PM?

Yes. Come alone.

Jacob went through the *Arizona Times Herald* internal messaging system and responded to sixteen questions about the next day's edition. At 2:30, he shut down his computer, picked up his backpack and left the building. After he arrived at the Marriott, he drove past it and parked in the Grenadine Ford's lot on the east side. A light sprinkle pestered his windshield, so he hurried across 57th street, circled around to a locked metal door on the side of the hotel and waited under the eave. Within a few minutes, a couple walked out and sprinted toward their car. He slipped inside the closing door, took the elevator to the third floor, and found room 346. He knocked lightly. After ten seconds of silence, he knocked again with more force. "Luca!" Hearing a door open behind him, he turned slowly to see a portly man part his blond bangs and wave him into room 347.

"Luca?"

"Yes. Come in. Hurry."

Jacob entered, and Luca closed the door behind him, locked the deadbolt, and secured the latch. "Not taking any chances, I see. Why the behavior?"

Luca motioned for Jacob to have a seat on one of two bamboo chairs while he sat in the other. "It would appear we both might be equally judicious," Luca smiled. "I watched your entrance into the hallway from my window."

Jacob grinned and nodded. "We can't be too careful." He was not going to open a conversation Luca had orchestrated, so he sat back and slung his arm over the back of the chair. "Oh, sorry to ask, but the clock on the wall behind you." Luca turned to see the clock he had not noticed before. "Would you mind if I turn it around?"

Luca gave him a puzzled look, then said, "Feel free, but I must ask what this is about."

"Thanks," said Jacob as he rose to cross the room and rotate the clock to face the wall. "It's a long story, but the short version is I've had a visceral reaction to clocks since I was a teenager. I think better without one in sight."

The real story was one he never shared with anyone. When he was eleven, he walked into the family bathroom to find his older brother dead in the bathtub. He had dropped an electric clock into the water. Though he looked up to a brother three years his senior, the fourteen-year-old was troubled. Jacob was too young to understand at the time, but later learned he was gay, and in 1991, gay was unacceptable at his school, at the family's Methodist church and within the Potter family. With no one to turn to, he decided things had to be better on the other side of life. Jacob knew someday he might have to allow a therapist to peel back the layers, but for now, avoiding clocks put an effective bandage on his past.

Jacob returned to his seat and said, "Now you may begin."

Luca wore maroon sweatpants and his plain gray T-shirt, which stretched over a well-padded paunch, showed sweat signs at the collar. His feet were bare and exposed calloused heels. Jacob recognized the disquieted voice with the Italian accent who had called the week before. "I have been reading your paper for the last month."

"Do you mind if I take notes?" Jacob asked.

"If you wish, but I do not think you will struggle with remembering facts."

"Nevertheless." Jacob reached inside his backpack and withdrew a notepad. "Your English seems to have improved dramatically in the last seven days, Mr. Luca. Is that what I call you?"

"Luca is fine. Before we start, may I see some identification, please?"

"Of course." Jacob withdrew his wallet and produced a business card from the *Arizona Times Herald*. "On the phone, your English was broken. Without your Venetian accent, I wouldn't have recognized your voice."

"Just being careful, Mr. Potter."

"Call me Jacob."

"Jacob it is. May I keep the card?"

"Please do, and feel free to continue." Jacob poised his pen above the paper. His memory was impeccable in earlier years, but over the last ten, there was a noticeable decline. He rationalized it had much more to do with age than his appreciation for fine cognacs. He learned to lean on his notes if for no other reason than to have tangible proof when he doubted himself.

Luca used his arms and hands like a paintbrush when he talked, assuming those in his audience needed illustrations to inhale his message completely. "This goes back to the year 1999 when a man named Enzo Caputo and I worked together in a genetics lab in Verona. It was his father's lab, and Enzo used some pull to get me in. We were the best of friends. The general manager disliked the fact we had what he felt was an easy . . . do you say avenue?"

"I understand."

"He assigned to us what he thought was a dead end . . . the field of prion diseases."

Jacob jerked his head up. "Now you have my attention."

"There was nothing sexy about them, but little was known, and we were attracted to them for that reason. We were only grad students at the time, but since the researchers saw little reason to use their resources on mysterious prions, they gave us free reign. We were even allowed to create our own hypotheses. The budget was meager, but we didn't need much."

Jacob felt good about bringing his pad. "I know a bit about the history of prions. There were a few committed researchers in the '90s who spent years in some very secluded and primitive tribes. Did you have much contact with these early researchers?"

"Only sporadically. Remember, we were just grad students, but we were true lab rats. Those guys liked to travel among the natives. That takes a different skill set."

"I see. Go on." Jacob shifted in his chair.

"If I may ask, how do you know about prion research?"

"We'll discuss that later. Promise, but continue your story."

"One of the unknowns at the time involved routes of transmission. Turns out there were multiple, but we concentrated on methods of airborne transmission. We were given the temporal lobe of the brain of a victim of Kuru, which, at the time, was transmitted through the endocannibalistic practices of the Fore tribe. They believed eating the brains of the deceased would return the life force of the deceased to the tribe."

"I've read about that community," said Jacob. "It's just a shade more difficult to understand than why my wife wears high heels to a Suns game."

Without acknowledging Jacob's attempt at humor, Luca

continued. "We also were given some brain tissue from an FFI victim they had in a sealed jar. Sorry, FFI stands for—"

"Fatal familial insomnia." Jacob grinned.

"You've done your homework, Jacob. Our hypothesis was diseased prions could also be transmitted through respiratory pathways. We experimented with frogs, especially *Xenopus tropacalis* or the African clawed frog because it's a diploid, just as most mammals are, including us."

"Sounds like a rare breed," said Jacob.

"Actually, it wasn't difficult to obtain them; they've been studied since 1940, even using them in pregnancy tests. South Africa breeds and exports them in ship loads."

"But diploid? What's that?"

"It just means they have two copies of each gene, one from the father and one from the mother. Our experiments were very rudimentary. Remember, our budget didn't allow for any expensive equipment. We used an enclosed incubator and blew a fan across the brain which sat in a sieve on top. There was a vacuum embedded in the floor which took the air and delivered it to containers which were later buried."

"Any rules on burying diseased prions at that time?"

"Like anything mysterious . . . think of AIDS in the eighties, there was fear. In fact, when someone died of a prion disease, they buried them in nine-foot graves. Not sure what those extra few feet provided other than more of a chance to introduce prions to the water table, but they didn't ask me."

Jacob was very familiar with the initial fear that surrounded AIDS. He and Dr. Kyle Hunter joined forces to educate the public thirty-five years ago. "Nine feet is nothing. In the eighties, they buried AIDS victims fourteen feet deep, and wouldn't even bury them in a cemetery."

Luca shook his head. "This is why I like research. To quote Sherlock Holmes, 'It is a capital mistake to theorize before one has data.' Anyway, at first, the fan was unable to transmit the prions to the frogs. We knew symptoms would show up in days . . . much faster than in humans. It's why we chose those guys. We had given up until Enzo thought of using different scents instead of just room air. He became obsessed."

Enzo took after his father, who would become so consumed with his work he would go days on amphetamines so he could avoid the great interrupter for a scientist: sleep.

"We blew every scent from Este Lauder perfume to garlic. Literally hundreds of scents. The air in the incubator was cleansed after seven days once we saw no symptoms and a new scent was used. We had to switch out frogs many times because we didn't want to mistake prion death for natural death. After almost three years, trying both Kuru and FFI tissues, we finally found the scent. When we dissected the frogs, we found the FFI prion proteins in the brains of the frogs. Just three out of the five died, by the way."

"I'm dying to know," Jacob said, realizing his accidental pun could have offended Luca. It didn't.

"It was vetivert oil."

"Not even sure what that is, but I've done a lot of research on these prions and never came across anything like this."

"I'm getting to that—"

"Wait, can you spell vetivert for me?"

After spelling it out, Luka added, "It comes from the vetiver plant. They make a French perfume out of it called Kus Kus."

"Never knew couscous was a perfume."

"If you're taking notes on this, Kus Kus is two words."

"Got it." Jacob was not sure what to do with this information, but made a note of it, anyway.

"And the reason only three died?" Luca asked, with curious eyebrows. He hesitated to see if Jacob cared about the trivial. When he didn't show much of a facial expression either way, he continued. "Collinge was doing some work with sporadic CJD sufferers and then Mad Cow at the time and postulated why some contract a prion disease and die while others show no symptoms—don't even get infected—is due to whether or not they were homozygous or heterozygous."

"This sounds like a biology lesson."

"Hang in there, Jacob. In a homozygote, they have an amino acid called valine in a key spot on each of their two prion genes. Keep in mind you and I, and almost every other mammal, has two copies of every gene. One from dad and one from mom."

"Makes us diploid, right?"

"See? You don't need to take notes. A heterozygote in my example has valine on only one prion gene and methionine on the other copy. He found with both CJD—that's Creutzfeldt-Jakob Disease and with BSE or Mad Cow, the homozygotes were far more likely to become infected. Just a few years before we did our research, Lugaresi and Gambetti considered this phenomenon in FFI and found the homozygotes were dying more rapidly while heterozygotes . . . well, their diseases were prolonged. I'm not sure what's worse."

Jacob could see a story forming now, but more importantly, information which could move the needle on solving the InF puzzle. "From what I'm hearing, and the numbers are growing from all over the country, the victims are all going through a short disease duration compared to FFI victims, or I suppose the majority of them, so are they all homozygotes?"

"Too early to tell. This is very new, as you know. We may be dealing with a prion which is different enough that it *only* affects homozygotes, who progress rapidly, or perhaps we're only hearing about the victims who die quickly. The good news is evolutionary forces have done a hatchet job on the homozygotes, because there are far more heterozygotes in every population than homozygotes. D.T. Max, in his book *The Family That Couldn't Sleep*, goes into hominid cannibalism to explain this, but no need for a history lesson right now."

"I may have to pick that up," Jacob said. "I never pass up a good cannibal story."

Not appreciating Jacob's humor, he continued. "There's also some newer research involving the zebrafish."

"Don't think I've seen that on any menus."

"Probably because their brains are much like ours—just simpler."

"I'm not taking the bait on that one."

"Huh?"

"Never mind. Go on."

"Anyway, they've shown if you depress or limit the DNA rebuilding protein called PARP1, the body doesn't sleep. Think about potholes in highways. When is the best time to fix these?"

Jacob enjoyed this exercise. "I suppose in the middle of the night when there's less traffic."

"Exactly how PARP1 works. It's like the construction engineer who works all day dealing with other headaches, then instructs night supervisors to get a crew and fix the holes on East Lebanon. If the engineer is out sick that day, the late shift workers go to a club and get little done because they don't know where the holes are."

"This is typical of the American workforce. When the cat's away, the mice will play."

"Great metaphor. May I use it?"

"It's all yours, Luca."

"Like the engineer, PARP1 is active during the day but before it retires, it sets in motion the DNA repair instructions for all components, but sleep is necessary to accomplish this due to less mental traffic. If you suppress PARP1, the zebrafish does not sleep. My theory is the folded proteins we see in FFI also include the PARP1 protein, much like tying up and gagging the engineer so he can't give instructions."

Jacob felt brain dead from the molecular overload. "PARPs and zebras aside, what happened next back in Veneto?"

"As I mentioned, Enzo's father ran the lab. When our discovery went up the chain of command, his father was kidnapped. Some of the events from those days are unclear, but what I *do* know is Enzo was forced to help an organization who wanted our data. He was moved to the U.S., and what he did was so secret that all communication between us immediately stopped. I received a letter from a strange address in Nebraska." He unfolded a piece of paper and held it up to read.

"You don't know me, but I write on behalf of Enzo Caputo. You will receive a call from him every Sunday at 9 a.m. MST, but you must not say anything. You are to connect the call, wait for the code phrase 'Sorry, incorrect number,' then quickly disconnect. If he ever fails to call you, you are to contact the *Arizona Times Herald* and report his death.

"And that is what you've done," Jacob said.

"Yes. Last Sunday, no call came. I didn't trust giving you details over the phone and for whatever reason, they've left me alone all these years. Right now, I don't believe that will continue."

Jacob stopped writing and regarded Luca. "Do you have any idea who was behind this?"

"I wish I knew. I could make some educated guesses, but they would likely be wrong. At every step, they've been invisible."

Jacob considered the gravity of Luca's statement. "What is your plan now? Are you going back to Italy?"

Luca shook his head, then mindlessly scanned the room. "I haven't decided. I want to explore what happened to my good friend. Enzo was a good person. He didn't deserve this. I want to avenge him, but I must consider the cost."

"Are you sure Enzo is dead? Maybe he's sick in a hospital. Maybe he lost his phone and didn't have your number memorized. Maybe he's just being held against his will somewhere." Jacob waited for a response which came slowly.

"You are grasping at straws. Do you know where that idiom came from?" he asked.

"No, but I suspect you do. Does it have anything to do with straws packed too tightly in a cannister, making it difficult to grab one?"

"Good try, but it was first mentioned in 1534 when Thomas More wrote in *Dialog of Comfort Against Tribulation*. He was referring to a drowning man who was grasping at anything to save himself, even the least likely object to help him."

"Thanks for the idiom lesson, Luca. But back to Enzo. Do you have proof he's dead?"

Luca shook his head. "I don't have proof, but I am very sure he's been killed. It's now been a week since he went silent. There is no scenario where I would not have heard from him by now. He had my number memorized. We couldn't trust him calling from his cell and we didn't want my number in his phone to connect us if it turned up in the wrong hands. If he was alive, he could have found a phone to call me. Anyone holding him would have eliminated him by now if they were trying to extract information. If they were holding him for ransom, we would have heard something by now and before you ask, I monitor the police traffic in both the Phoenix area and Montana. Besides, knowing what I know, there would be no reason to hold him for ransom. They would have simply killed him."

"Does he have any family?" Jacob asked.

"Yes. He is married."

Jacob sighed. "And she knows nothing, I assume."

"We will never know."

"What does that mean? What happened?" Jacob straightened in his chair.

"His wife and her mother died in a house fire two nights ago. As I said, I monitor the police communication in Montana, and I knew his wife's name. The fire was ruled accidental, but I know the truth."

42

Release Authorization

Phoenix Department of Environmental Management. On July 7, 2021, an Accident Investigation Board was appointed to investigate an explosion which occurred on July 6, 2021 at 2:07 p.m. MST at the Shanghai Dry Cleaners on 5647 Bell Road. The Board's responsibilities have been completed with respect to this investigation. The analysis and the identification of the contributing causes, the root cause and the Judgments of Need resulting from this investigation were performed in accordance with DOE Order 225.1B, Accident Investigations.

The report of the Accident Investigation Report has been accepted and the authorization to release this report for general distribution has been granted.

Madden Wilder

Madden Wilder
Deputy Assistant Secretary
Safety, Security, and Quality Programs
Office of Environmental Management

"That's Antioch," said Poseidon. He punched the red button.

"Has it been cleaned up?" the gravelly voice on the phone asked.

"Yes. The Salamander needs the other half wired. When he gets the money, he'll send the coordinates where we can locate the body. His usual MO. All we know is he had left Arizona."

"I'll take care of it. Still don't like the way he handled the laundry. Too messy."

"That's been taken care of," said Poseidon. "It's been logged as an accidental explosion. We need the Salamander anymore?"

"If he'll stay until the twenty-third, we might use him on another job. Tell him to . . . never mind. I'll handle him from my end. How is our man on the inside at the *Arizona Times Herald*? Anything to report?"

"Not yet. He's working a few angles, but he has to keep a low profile."

"And the site? Anything to worry about?"

Poseidon hesitated. "We received a letter from the BBB, but nothing serious. It was expected, and we've handled it."

Without a word, Antioch ended the call. Poseidon turned to Falcon. "You think he knows about Quito's escape?"

Falcon shook his head. "I don't know how, but nothing would surprise me. He's got eyes in the back of his head. That was a cluster. I wasn't ready to tell him. We need to get that cleaned up yesterday."

"We're working on it. Several dead ends but one lead sounds promising. I'll let you know." Poseidon walked out the side door onto the gravel path, which led to the helipad where his pilot had the red piper spinning. He climbed in, and the bird soon disappeared over Camelback Mountain.

43

The sun snuck over the eastern peak and casted early morning shadows of a deer blind across the breakfast table on Kyle's back patio. As Kristy cleared away the dishes, he pulled Marie aside to discuss the YMCA meeting, which was slated for the evening. "I'm hoping to get some answers tonight. It's like officials have blinders on. My patients trust me, and I trust them, so maybe we'll discover something."

She peered up at him and shielded her eyes from the sun. "After what's been happening, this makes me nervous, Kyle. If you're in a large group of people searching for the source of this pandemic, and if forces beyond our control are intent on stopping that, it could get real. Have you considered hiring some enforcement officers?"

He shook his head. "I'm afraid that could send a signal. Like to stay under the radar. You're welcome to come, but I'd strongly oppose it."

"Then I'm not welcome." She smiled.

Kyle grinned. "Just a southerner's way of softening the blow."

Marie had let her office know she was taking a few days off, but she felt helpless and stagnant in this hideaway on the east side of the McDowell Mountains. "Although I think you're crazy, I also think you're brave. The plan's good, but I would put the threat level at somewhere between 'wear body armor' and 'hide in an underground bomb shelter.' I think I'll pass and take your bike for a ride this evening if you don't mind."

"Not at all," Kyle said as he stood. "Kristy has an Aventon Pace 500, which might work better for you, especially if you'll be climbing the mountain. She hasn't ridden but once since I bought it for her."

"Sounds great. It'll give me some time to think. And to *not* think about the risk you're taking. I'd like to get in twenty miles."

"I'll lay out a thermal jersey and some shorts for you, along with some shoes. If Kristy's don't fit, and they should, but if they don't, we have some of Katrina's here you can try. She's away at UCLA and left everything here."

"Thanks, Kyle."

The gentle cooing of white-winged doves drifted across the lake. In the distance, Kyle could see a doe and her fawn peeking out of some underbrush. His riding lawnmower sat idle to his left, perennial ryegrass overtaking the wheels, and a neglected vegetable garden next to it begged for some attention. *This must end soon*, he reflected. He walked in with Marie and Jilian, laid out some clothes for Marie, then excused himself to prepare for the meeting.

As Kristy loaded the dishwasher, Marie turned to Jilian. "I never got to meet the senator, but I could tell she was a very special person."

Jilian nodded. "Very special friend, as well. I miss her."

"You'll be carrying on for her? Do you know who'll be taking her place? I've not had time to follow politics, I'm afraid."

Jilian's thoughts took on a melancholy tone. "I feel helpless. Governor Adair was . . . well, I *thought* he was a friend of Senator Bonner, but after she died, he made no efforts to acknowledge her work. He didn't come to the funeral, and then he appointed Orlando Bradley over the senator's pick of Judge Stoutmeyer to carry on her work. It breaks my heart to see all her hard work scratched and dismembered."

"Is that the same Orlando Bradley who—"

"The very one. His daddy was a well-respected 9th circuit court judge and got him off the pornography charge."

"I'm so sorry." Marie had no words of wisdom. No expressions of comfort. She could work wonders with patients who presented with insomnia and a myriad of other sleep problems, but the machinations of government bodies were anathema to her.

After a short nap, Marie awoke to see Kyle had laid out everything she needed. She dressed, filled the water bottle, then pedaled seventy yards at an incline up Ponderosa Lane, wishing she had started her ride with less of a challenge. Her watch read 4:31. Before leaving, she mapped out a twenty-mile ride, which would include several repeated loops, and programmed the trip on her *Map My Ride* app.

This bike did not have the speed of her Trek-Segafredo, but it took the terrain without blinking. Nothing brought her blood pressure down more than riding through the wind. The afternoon sun was now at her back as she headed east on the Midlife Crisis trail. She chose this route because most hikers and bikers would have finished their day early to avoid the heat of the day, something she fed on. Swallowed it whole. This would give her more privacy. Sweat dripped from her brows but was quickly whisked away by the oncoming air currents.

She never knew why. Or maybe she did. Icarus was the character in her favorite Greek myth, so she had made a game of riding as close to tall Saguaro cacti as she could without getting stuck. On every ride, she would inch closer and closer to these until she felt the needles scratch the side of her jersey. On one of these pass-bys, she whisked by a few hikers who watched this exercise with disbelief.

She was alone again as the sun inched its way westward. After a few miles, she could hear the low hum of motorcycle engines in the distance. She thought at first, they must be driving along the highway, but soon realized the sounds were getting closer. As she rode into a clearing, she rubbernecked and could see smoke billowing in the distance. She knew motorcycles were not allowed on these trails, and her pulse quickened. One hundred yards ahead, she could see familiar large rock outcroppings. They were familiar, but she had never explored their anatomy.

She doubled her pace, crouching low against the bar. The sweat no longer evaporated. Her jersey was damp. The cycle sounds grew closer, and she could now hear the revving of two separate engines. As she made it to the rock formations, she found a narrow opening between two large rocks which were rooved by a larger one. It appeared as if it had dropped out of the sky, or rolled down the mountain, and wedged between the two. She rode through and angled left, spotted a small cave, then dropped her bike and considered calling 911, but thought it best to maintain silence for now. She ran inside the cave to discover hundreds of Karst crickets running helter-skelter across the ceiling. She shivered as she crouched lower to listen. As the motorcycles drew close, they slowed and stopped, idling in neutral thirty feet from the cave entrance. Through a crack between two boulders, she could see two helmeted riders with opaque visors.

They sat for what felt to Marie like minutes until a husky male voice said, "Dr. Jimmerson, this is to illustrate we know where you are . . . always . . . but you are to mention this to no one. We will know if you do not respect our position. Do you acknowledge?"

Marie sat quiet and considered not speaking. She could see a familiar mark on the slender wrist of one rider as a jacket sleeve rode up their forearm.

"If you do not acknowledge, we will be forced to come in there and drag you out."

"I acknowledge!" she yelled shakily, trying her best to recall where she had seen the mark.

A female voice said, "Alton and Jean have a very nice home in Tampa Bay."

Marie shivered as she thought of her parents in harm's way. They rode away as quickly as they had arrived. Her heartbeat refused to slow. It felt like she was riding uphill with no relief in sight. She laid down on her back, closed her eyes, and prayed.

44

Accident and Investigation Board Report,
Phoenix Department of Environmental Management:
Executive Summary.

On Tuesday, July 6, 2021, at approximately 02:07 p.m. Mountain Standard Time, an explosion occurred at the Shanghai Dry Cleaners on 5647 Bell Road, Phoenix. There were three adults in the building when the explosion occurred. Two were treated on-site for smoke inhalation, then transported to Banner Hospital (BH). One was fatally injured at the site and another succumbed to injuries at BH. On July 7, 2021, Madden Wilder, Deputy Assistant Secretary for Safety, Security, and Quality Programs, U.S. Department of Energy, Office of Environmental Management formally appointed an Accident Investigation Board (the Board) to investigate the accident in accordance with DOE Order (O) 225.1B, based on this accident meeting Accident Investigation Criteria 2.d.1 of DOE O 225.1B, Accident Investigations, Appendix A. The Board began the investigation on July 8, 2021, completed the investigation on July 10, 2021, and submitted findings to the Deputy Assistant Secretary for Safety, Security, and Quality Programs Environmental Management on July 11, 2021. The Board concluded this accident was preventable.

Accident Description: The explosion is believed to have originated in the IT closet of Shanghai Dry Cleaners, which had been closed for over three months. A slow gas leak from a broken seal in the line to one of the industrial dryers provided the environmental backdrop. A rusted pea trap holding some fluid in an upstairs kitchen leaked through the ceiling, shorting out the server in the downstairs closet, igniting the gas. The explosion, although begun in the IT closet, made the air throughout the building combustible within milliseconds. Two nearby walkers sustained minor injuries but were the first ones on the scene to survey the damage. They assisted in helping free the victim who survived. It remains unknown as to why the three victims were in the closed building and as to why the gas was not turned off when the business closed during the COVID pandemic. Efforts at contacting the surviving victim proved unsuccessful.

Kyle drove to the YMCA and planned to be there thirty minutes early to set up, but there were more than fifty vehicles in the parking lot at 6:30 on July 14.

"Jiminy Cricket!"

He walked inside and noticed there were many faces he did not recognize, but the smell and lack of efficient air conditioning were remarkably familiar. Squeaking tennis shoes and perspiration combined to penetrate the wooden stands. No amount of disinfectant could, or should, mask the past.

Toby Fairchild approached him first, oil-stained hand extended. "Hey, Doc. I couldn't help but notice a face wracked with confusion when you walked in. I figured either you forgot where you was or saw some folks you don't know."

"I was that transparent?" he asked, feeling unclothed.

"You telegraphed it right nicely. A bunch o' your patients brung their kith and kins. You may just get a buttload o' new patients from this here town hall meetin'! Sorry. Didn't mean to use that French."

"It's okay, Toby. Getting new patients is not my goal tonight, but I'm glad to see so many here. I think I'll break everyone up into groups of ten for some table discussions. Can you help me set up some tables?"

"Sure thing, Doc. Hey John! Carl! Help us out!"

After more than three hundred arrived by a few minutes after seven and found seats at one of thirty-five tables, Kyle took the mic. "Thank you all for coming out this evening. Let me first say I've been praying for all of you who are suffering or will suffer with the insomnia flu. The goal of this evening is to unearth a common denominator . . .anything at all which binds the InF community together. It is my belief that once we discover the root cause, catalyst, or instigator behind this awful disease, we will be that much closer to a cure, or perhaps a vaccination."

A round of applause, though tepid, rewarded his comments.

"You will notice I placed papers on your table—one for each of you. I'd like you to answer the questions privately, and after ten minutes, you are to compare and discuss among your table. You will then elect a captain who will stand and let us know if you found any commonalities. Any questions?" Seeing none, he said, "Great! Get to work!"

He wandered around the room as they wrote and noted everyone was in his or her own specific stage of disrepair. Some were lethargic, unable to create a thought to put down on paper. Some were in pain, and a good number of nurturers drew energy by helping a suffering partner. After ten minutes, he told them to start the discussion. Again, as he worked the room, he recognized some who could not talk, but were writing on paper anything they wanted to communicate. He knew those attendees did not have long to live.

1. Do you have symptoms of the insomnia flu?
2. Have you had any cooked food delivered to your place of residence in the last year?
3. Do you own any animals? If so, what kind(s)?
4. Do you have allergies? If so, to what?
5. Have you had the flu shot regularly?
6. Have you received anything unexpectedly in the mail?
7. Have you had your air conditioning system or water heater worked on within the last year?
8. Do you drink bottled water?
9. Name any plants you have inside your home.
10. Since you turned fifty, have you eaten anything new, and if so, what was it?
11. Since turning fifty, have you been prescribed a new medication? If so, what was it?

It was a raucous group, with the volume slowly escalating to a pitch which would rival a discussion on funding an after-school program by the PTA. Kyle had to raise his voice, then blow a whistle into the mic to get the group to calm down.

A hand toward the back of the room waved frantically. "Peter's got something to say," Kyle said. "Go ahead. . . and use your outside voice so all can hear."

Nan ran a portable mic over to him as he started speaking.

"Four of us have golden doodles!" There was some general murmuring, some holding up their hands and saying various versions of, "Me too!"

"Do you all have InF symptoms?" Kyle asked.

Peter said, "Only two of us." Another hand raised to indicate he was a doodle owner and had symptoms.

"Thanks, Peter." As he panned the crowd, he asked, "Anyone else come up with some interesting coincidences?" A hand in the back raised from a woman he did not recognize. "Yes? What did you uncover?"

The middle-aged plump blonde stood, waited on the mic from Nan and said, "We have four at our table who had the flu shot and all of us have symptoms of the insomnia flu."

"All right," said Kyle. "Now we're getting somewhere. All of you who have had the flu shot regularly, stand up." About two-thirds stood, some hesitantly as they didn't know how to define *regularly,* and some painstakingly. "Now, everyone with symptoms, please sit down. About half took a seat. "You may be seated. I know this isn't scientific and don't take any of this to the bank, but so far, I'm not impressed enough to take anything further." A lady to his left who wore an Arizona Cardinals' ball cap, raised her hand. "Yes, Melinda?"

She stood and took the mic. "We don't have them anymore, but most of us had a plant mailed to us about twenty years ago for our thirtieth birthday. None of us remember who it was from, but everyone remembers it smelled amazing.

Kyle froze when the room erupted with shouts of "I got that plant back then!" and "I remember that plant!" There were a few who said they had given theirs away. The tenor of the room continued to rise until Kyle spoke into the mic.

"Let's see a show of hands. Who recalls getting this plant mailed to them twenty years ago?" Over ninety percent of the room raised their hands, some of them both hands to make sure they were counted. The scene brought a collective gasp within the gym. He spoke again, "Does anyone remember any details at all about who sent it or where it came from? Who delivered it? Anything would help. Nothing is too trivial."

No one spoke. No one raised their hands. He could tell most were deep in thought, rubbing small round circles on their temples. Some gazed at the water-stained ceiling and others had their heads bowed in a prayer-like pose.

After a minute, a woman named Starlene jumped out of her chair and said, "It was something like Best News! I remember thinking that was rather ironic since I was turning thirty-three, the same age Jesus was when he was crucified, and the world was about to end for me, too." This begat more murmurings and handwringing. A feeble man near Kyle tried to stand but found it difficult.

Kyle walked over, placed a hand on his shoulder to signal him to stay seated and asked, "Do you want to tell us something, Vince?"

He held the mic down to his mouth. "I remember something about horizons. Maybe best new horizons?"

"Brand New Horizons!" came a high-pitched voice from his left. The congregational nodding of heads that ensued reminded Kyle of playing Whack-A-Mole.

Vince said, "That's it! Brand New Horizons!"

Kyle felt energized. "So, you're all saying either a company named Brand New Horizons sent you this plant?" More nodding and verbal affirmations. "Or," he continued, "could it have been the message you received and not the name of the sender?" Considerable chatter raised the volume level again as they argued the distinction.

After a minute, Kyle asked, "How many of you think it was the name of the company?" A scattering of hands lifted. "All right, now how many of you think it was the message?" Only two hands. "Okay, folks," Kyle continued. "You have been most helpful. I'll continue to pray for you as we travel this obscure road together. Have a good evening!"

Although Kyle had been on edge enough to scan the room repeatedly and look for anyone suspicious, he wanted to leave the building in a group, reasoning if anyone wished to do him harm, they would not choose to do so in a crowd. This would not be difficult, as about fifteen surrounded him currently to ask questions or to thank him for the evening. "Should I throw away my plant? Hope you and the police catch those pricks! Hey, doc, you having any InF symptoms? This what this is all about?"

"No, Tim, not at all. I hate seeing my patients going through this. It's miserable and I'm doing my best to help find out more information."

"Dr. Kyle! My name is Cindy Portillo. I'm not a patient of yours but—"

Kyle's attention moved to a man he failed to recognize, but who stood with his arms crossed leaning against the collapsed bleachers. Younger than anyone at the meeting, he wore a blond ascot hat which matched a full beard, and he concentrated on a cell phone.

"I'm sorry, Ms. Portillo. My attention took a vacation. Something my wife's gotten used to. You were saying?"

"I was saying in the eighties, I was a member of the Zero Population Group and through the years, a radical faction—"

Another man walked up to the bearded interloper, and they began talking. They were a good sixty feet away, so Kyle could not hear anything, but uneasiness controlled him. With his pulse quickening, he turned again to Ms. Portillo, and said, "I'm so sorry, but I've been needing to use the restroom since I got here. Will you excuse me?"

He didn't wait for her response but walked as casually as he could toward the bathroom area in the rear of the gym. Once inside, he looked for an exterior window. No luck. He walked into a stall and sat on the commode lid to think.

"Nan."

He texted her.

> Don't ask why but please find the fire alarm and
> set it off. Then come stand by the men's bathroom
> door and if someone tries to enter, make them go
> outside. I saw Toby and some others still hanging
> around if you need help.

She texted back.

> I got this.

Thirty seconds later, the alarm went off. It was deafening even
inside the bathroom. He could hear yelling and general commotion, but it was difficult to hear much above the discordant whine.
In a few minutes, he heard sirens. They were getting louder, but
then started to recede. A knock at the door caused him to jump.

"Dr. Hunter?"

Kyle left the stall and stood next to the sink. "Everything
copacetic out there, Nan?"

She responded with a raised voice. "Yes, everyone has left the
gym, but some are just standing around outside. Can I just come
in or are you coming out?"

"All clear in here. Come in so we can talk."

Nan walked through the door with a puzzled look. "What's
going on?"

"Did you see two younger guys? One blond with a beard and
another with a moustache and—"

"Yes. Good thing you told me about Toby. They were headed
to this bathroom, and he moved them along. Probably helps he's
a dead ringer for a Hell's Angel. John and Carl were with him, so
they didn't object too much."

Kyle leaned against the sink cabinet and braced his chin in his right hand. After a few thoughtful seconds, he asked, "Hey, I just remembered the sirens. What happened to the firemen?"

"Hmm . . . now that you bring that up, I did see the young guy with the moustache make a call on his cell, and about two minutes later, the sirens went away. I wonder—"

"That's what I was afraid of," said Kyle. "I haven't filled you in on everything, but some people have been hurt. Some killed. I don't know what's going on, but we have to be careful."

"Why would anyone want to hurt you? Or us? Are you sure you're not being paranoid?" Nan had not seen this side of Kyle in the thirty years they had worked together.

"It's too early to tell, Nan, but on the surface, it looks like anyone connected with finding out more about the insomnia flu is in danger. Dr. Jimmerson felt uneasy about tonight. Maybe I shouldn't have—"

"No, Dr. Hunter. Your efforts tonight might play a big part in solving this mess. I—"

"Wait," Kyle said as he edged away from the counter and stood. "Do you know when those two guys came in? Did you see them during the meeting?"

Nan thought for a few seconds and investigated her memory bank which held the last ninety minutes. "I walked all around the gym with that mic, and I don't remember them at all."

"Good," Kyle said emphatically. "Maybe they didn't hear what we learned."

"Unless they had a spy in there who called them during the meeting," Nan offered.

Kyle frowned. "I didn't need that. Can you walk outside and pretend to talk to some of our patients but look around for those guys? Most might be headed home already so we can't waste any more time. We need to leave as a group."

"I'll be right back." Nan twirled and headed back through the bathroom door. She peeked around the corner and peered through the glass entry doors toward the parking lot and saw no movement. She walked slowly and looked back and forth as she approached the doors.

"Nan! Come back!" Kyle walked out of the bathroom and motioned her to return. As she hurried back, the glass shattered behind her, and the shock threw her to the floor. Kyle rushed over and saw she was dazed but awake. He dragged her back through the bathroom door. "That was a bullet," he said breathlessly as he managed to get the door closed behind her and lock it. "Now do you believe me?"

"That door won't stop bullets, Kyle!"

"It's okay. I called 911 before I yelled for you and told them there was a break-in at the Y. I hear the police coming now. Now I'm glad that door is blown apart. They'll be ready when they get here." Kyle looked down to see blood pooling from under Nan. "Hey, turn over."

"What?"

"Just do it." When she turned to her stomach, he saw the piece of glass lodged in her back. "Good grief, Nan. Do you not feel this glass sticking out of your back?"

"It does sting some, but I kinda got thrown to the floor, so I wasn't sure what I was feeling."

"All right. I'm removing it, and then I'm going to apply direct pressure to stop the bleeding until someone comes. Should be soon. Besides, since you're wounded, they'll know we aren't the bad guys."

After he removed it and applied pressure, Nan said, "Thanks doctor. Sorry I called you Kyle. Very unprofessional of me."

Kyle shook his head and as he did, they heard voices through the door. "Anyone in here? Anyone? Chuck! There's a bullet!"

They could hear two men drop to the floor and begin crawling. "You take the hall! I'll head this way!"

After a minute, Kyle figured it best to open the door and get their attention. Nan's bleeding had subsided, and he rolled her over so the pressure of the floor could continue to stem any flow.

He slowly opened the door, but after a few inches, a voice said, "Hands only! Stick both of your hands out the door! I have a gun trained on you right now, so don't try anything!"

Kyle protruded both arms through the door as he said, "I am Dr. Kyle Hunter and I have a bleeding woman in here. She was hurt when the shot went through the door. May I come out?"

"Yes," the officer said, "but keep your hands out."

Kyle walked out with his hands high. "She needs medical attention. I don't have what she needs on me, so we need to get her to the hospital."

"Sir. Dr. Hunter. Do you know if there is anyone else in the building?"

"I can't promise, but I don't think so."

"How bad is she?" he asked as he stood and faced Kyle.

"Not that bad, and before you ask, we hid in there from whoever was out there attempting to do us harm."

Officer Fields grinned. "Of course. We didn't see any cars leaving as we drove up."

"Your siren probably scared them away. At least I hope so."

"Any idea who would do this?" Fields asked as he withdrew a pad and pen.

"I have no idea. We were just having a meeting here and—"

"I thought the Y was closed. Was this a legal event?"

Kyle wrinkled his eyebrows. "Listen, I need to get Nan out of that bathroom and to the hospital. Can we continue the interrogation later? I assure you it was a legal meeting. You can check with the city manager. His name is Braxton—"

"Yes, I know the city manager, Dr. Go ahead and get your friend. We'll follow you to the hospital."

Kyle started toward the bathroom, but turned and said, "Don't you have to report this? Someone shot at us, for crying out loud."

"Chuck already called it in. We have forensics and an investigator coming out."

"Seems excessive, Officer Fields."

"Treating it as a hate crime. Someone hates glass doors. Now go get your lady."

Kyle smirked and headed through the bathroom door. He emerged a minute later, carrying Nan. "You know what? I've got sutures and dressing at the house. I think I'll just take her there. Braxton has my number so call me and we can discuss any other details later. He walked carefully through glass shards and out the door toward his car.

Fields called after him. "What was the meeting about?" But Kyle was gone.

45

Marie rode into Kyle's driveway, once she had somewhat recovered emotionally from the encounter with the motorcycle riders. It was close to 9:00 p.m. and Kyle met her at the door.

"We were worried about you. Why weren't you answering your phone?"

She was prepared for the questioning. "Phone ran out of juice. Forgot to charge it. Sorry!" She dismounted and wheeled the bike inside as Kyle opened the door. "I've got to get a shower. We can talk more in twenty minutes."

"Take your time. There's some lasagna in the oven. Help yourself. I've got to make a call."

As she showered, she wondered how, or even if, she should deflect Kyle's questions. She punched in as many variables as she could, doing her best to dissect the message of the riders. Was there a connection to the explosion? Was she getting too close with her prion questioning? Was anyone else in danger? She concluded, for now, she would keep this event to herself.

Darkness interrupted only by a harvest moon greeted Kyle

through his arched window as he walked into his office and tapped Jacob's number.

"Hello, Dr. Hunter. I hope this is important. Word of warning: the wife is sitting next to me and paused *Dancing With Stars* so I could answer this call from you."

"You know I wouldn't call this late if it wasn't important. I have some information for you on the insomnia flu which could help you and the authorities locate who's responsible."

Jacob excused himself from the living room couch and told Wendy to watch it without him. "Tell me more, Kyle."

"We held a town hall meeting tonight and—"

"Thanks for alerting me before it happened."

"All right, I deserved that, but it was a meeting I set up to talk to my patients in their fifties. No one else was invited, but my patients took it upon themselves to invite their friends. There were over three hundred packed into the YMCA gym."

"That's quite a turnout. Were you passing out doobies?"

"No, but it was about the insomnia flu, and that gets people turning out. Answers have been hard to come by these days, but long story short, about nine out of ten tonight received a plant back around the year 2000 when they turned thirty-three. With Y2K going on, they worried more about the world ending than what company was responsible for mailing them a plant."

"So did you get any answers?" Jacob asked.

"They were called Brand New Horizons, and don't bother searching online. Kristy and I searched, and we found no information at all. None. They disappeared into thin air."

"How sure are you Brand New Horizons is the correct name of the company?"

"Almost a hundred percent. Everyone who could still remember back twenty years."

"But these—"

"I know where you're going. Remember, this flu doesn't affect the memory until late in the disease timeline. These patients are thinking clearly, other than hallucinations, all the way to the end. Anyway, they all said that was the name. It took a little guesswork at first, but everyone agreed by the time the discussion was over."

"So, they got a plant from this Brand New Horizons company. What next?"

"That's your job. Oh, one lady—wait, I got her name right here . . . Jennifer Mata. She's a physician, by the way. One of those whole health types. Says she had the plant until a few weeks ago."

"That figures."

"She claims to have kept every plant given to her since she turned eighteen, but she ran out of room and traded it to the Bennington Nursery for some fertilizer. I figured we could get the police to investigate and see if there were any latent prints."

"From twenty years ago? Is that possible?"

"I'm no expert," Kyle said, "but I would bet they can be lifted if they haven't been rubbed off. If she's left it in her home in the same place for all those years, maybe?"

"Likely delivered by someone unrelated to the company, but we have to start somewhere," said Jacob. He could hear raucous clapping and familiar whistles from the living room and considered the timing of the interruption to be fortuitous, regardless of the subject. The fact this news could give a productive boost to his investigation was a bonus.

"Not sure what type of specialist would be needed to see if the plant could transmit the virus, or prion or—"

"Wait a minute, Doc," Jacob interrupted. "Dr. Jimmerson may be right."

"Yes. That's why I mentioned prions. Fatal familial insomnia takes decades to manifest into symptoms and few die before their fifties."

"Any other reason to specifically suspect FFI instead of other prion diseases?"

"Yes, Marie said it's the only known prion disease that's almost impossible to diagnose. Even the most specific test, the RT-QuIC, which has a 95% sensitivity and 100% specificity for other prion diseases does a poor job of diagnosing FFI."

"Marie's been holding out on me. Never heard of RT-QuIC. So, you think they chose FFI because they could hide the disease behind others?"

"Yes. Also, dementia is one of the *first* symptoms of all other prion diseases but only occurs in the latter stages of FFI, so symptoms are usually mistaken as signs of other pathologies. If I was going to slip in a prion disease on an unsuspecting public and wanted to delay the discovery for decades, I'd choose FFI."

"Have you thought out your next step?"

"I'm not even sure who to contact first. Not the police, but the CDC? The Feds? A local epidemiologist?"

"It's a crime scene, best I can tell," said Jacob.

"You're right."

"We just may run a piece in the morning, but we won't name names or provide any details we don't know. I appreciate the tip but need to run. I've got to get this in the right hands." He made the prudent decision not to mention what he learned from Luca.

"Oh, one more thing, Jacob. Someone fired a shot through the front door of the Y tonight when we were trying to leave."

Jacob paused before saying anything. "You waited this long to tell me?"

"I recounted the events chronologically, since you're taking notes."

"Anyone hurt? Police come?"

"Not bad. Nan took a piece of glass in the back, but I've got her bandaged up at the house. And yes, the police came because I called them." Kyle related the string of events, concluding with their exit.

Jacob digested the story, then said, "That was some type of warning. If they were trying to eliminate anyone, they could have shot Nan before you called her back or even waited until you were both outside and shot you both. I think you should consider yourself warned. Someone didn't like that you called that meeting."

"I agree," Kyle said. "You think it's related to the explosion that killed Danny?"

"Hard to say, but until I know more, we have to assume there's a connection. We also have to assume the two men know everything you learned, even though they didn't show up until later. Someone tipped them off."

Kyle shivered as he considered the danger he had invited in. Nan's injury, the danger to his wife Kristy, the warning which could turn into something more serious if not heeded. When he fought with Jacob in the days of AIDS, when his father fought the tobacco industry, nothing like this happened. Or perhaps it had, and he was oblivious. He would have to sleep on this and make some decisions tomorrow.

"If they meant to scare me from passing on what I learned, it didn't work. Now you know. Night, Jacob. I may have to take some trazodone to get to sleep myself." He removed the shotgun from his gun safe, locked all the doors, then checked them all again to make sure. After the alarm was set, he told Kristy, Jilian, and Marie they were leaving the lights on all night and decided he would let Marie fill him in on what happened on her ride when she was ready. She was keeping something from him, and after tonight, every detail needed investigating.

46

Sawyer hopped in the passenger's seat of the Tesla Model X, and it pulled away onto Fourth Street. Fog rolled in during the early morning hours and gave the wipers a signal to erase the leftovers. The sun threatened to erupt over Bridger Mountain and once again usher in a triple-digit offering. He often wondered how he would have adapted to a life in Green Bay, Wisconsin.

After his playing days at Oregon State as a free safety concluded, he was asked to be an assistant secondary coach for the Packers. They considered the cerebral Sawyer to be worthy of moving up the ranks after he served as a player/coach his senior year. He weathered the cold winters in the beaver state well, but Green Bay would be in another stratosphere, so he found a job in construction in the Phoenix area and put out feelers to warm-weather football programs which never materialized.

"Thanks for picking me up, Kira, but geez. 6:30? What's all the cloak and dagger about?"

His khakis appeared to have been rescued from the dirty clothes hamper and the gray T-shirt was pulled over a muscular frame created by daily trips to the gym. The two-day beard made him more attractive to Kira, but she knew any type of relationship with a coworker must remain platonic.

"Sorry I couldn't say more on the phone. This is hitting too close to home." She related to Sawyer their experience at the hospital, the guard at the door, their absconding with Jilian Quito and the holing up of her and Dr. Marie Jimmerson at Dr. Hunter's lake house. "Difficult time sleeping last night. I don't even feel safe in my own home." She drove along 303 without a destination in mind.

"If you're so scared, why didn't you stay secluded with them?"

"I couldn't do that. I have work to do. Have to carry on for Danny. We may not have liked him, but he didn't have to die."

"Kira, I think you're blowing this all out of proportion. The guard could have been—"

"You weren't there!" She gripped the steering wheel tighter and stared straight ahead. "You think the explosion that killed Danny was an accident?"

"We don't know anything yet. Could've been a water heater. It could've been—"

"But it wasn't," Kira said firmly. "Someone knew they were meeting there, and we don't know who it was meant for. Could have been Jilian Quito. Could have been Danny, and that's what concerns me most."

"What about Darcy Sandam? Maybe it was meant for her?"

"I thought about that, but it makes the least sense. She's just a widow with no ties to anyone who I can see." Kira said this with less conviction than she intended.

"So, if it really was a bomb meant to kill someone, and I still have my doubts . . . if it was meant for Danny, I can see your concern, but I see two holes in your theory. If it was meant for Danny, why was there a guard posted outside Jilian's room? Secondly, why would anyone want *him* dead? He's just an editor."

"We're reporters, Sawyer. Investigative reporters. We have to consider every possibility. You know that. I know the police are investigating, but right now, I don't know who to trust. Maybe Danny had uncovered something he wasn't supposed to. My question is, who knew that meeting would happen at that time and in that location?"

"Exactly," said Sawyer with emphasis. "It's why I think this will surface as an accidental explosion once the police are finished."

Kira shot him an accusatory glance. "If you don't want to help, that's fine, but I—"

"Wait, Kira. I didn't say I wouldn't help, but let's wait for some proof. So far, they've ruled it—"

"I know what they said, but I don't believe it."

"By the way, you'll want to hear this. I got a call this morning, even before you called me, by an anonymous caller. He wouldn't give me his name."

She exited the highway without turning on her indicator. "And?"

"He said he knew who still owned a plant and gave me a name and address."

"Why did he call *you*?"

"Because Jacob was gone and not answering his cell, Danny is . . . well . . . so they sent the message to me. I think we should go check it out."

"I consider the word of a person named *anonymous* with skepticism, and even if he's telling the truth, I'm not sure I want to be up close and personal with one of those plants, Sawyer."

"I have a mask, so I'll take care of it. I'll put it in the trunk, anyway. We need to get it to Throckmorton for evaluation. We need proof that what Dr. Hunter found in his town hall meeting is true."

"Throckmorton? Thought he was in Pittsburgh."

"Jacob financed his trip down and arranged for him to spend a few weeks on the paper's dime. He can be quite convincing, as you know."

"Yes, he can. Punch in the address." She pulled up to a charging station while Sawyer scrolled through his phone to his note on the address and typed it into the Tesla's GPS. "The charge can wait. I'd like to see about that plant." When they arrived twenty-five minutes later at the home on Cheshire Avenue, Sawyer walked through an unlocked, latched iron gate into an enclosed courtyard and knocked on a Tudor door with three vertical windows. From the car, Kira watched a door open, a short conversation with a blond who shook her ponytail from side to side and a return of Sawyer to the car.

"Says she didn't call and doesn't have the plant. Says she hates plants." He latched his seatbelt and took his phone out to inspect the text.

"Did you punch it in wrong?" asked Kira.

"Nope. It's correct. Checked three times. This is frustrating. Hey, my stomach is growling. Let's get some lunch. My treat."

She drove away from the plantless house. "I'm taking you home. Don't feel like eating right now anyway."

47

On the morning of July fifteenth, Jacob called Kyle. He had decided to pass on information he learned from Luca without implicating him or putting him in any danger.

"Sorry to bother you, but our preliminary research leads us to believe this insomnia flu could be contagious as well as infectious, so what you discovered from your patient base is appearing more believable." Jacob hoped he was not betraying Luca's confidence.

"I don't take any solace in this. It just means many more may die."

"That's why I'm calling. We've contacted Throckmorton—"

"The epidemiologist?"

Jacob could have sworn he heard an odd echo as Kyle spoke . . . the same peculiar sound from a conversation the other day with Marie. But he continued, ignoring the paranoid thoughts. "That's right. He would like to get one of the plants to the virology lab at ADHS to run some tests. You said one of your patients still owned a plant?"

"Yes. Her name is Barbara Harvey. Let me get her contact information for you." He clicked a few tabs in his EMR, then said, "Tell you what. Just so there's no confusion, let me text you her number and address. I'm guessing you're not involving the police yet?"

"You guessed right. However, I can't tell *you* not to go to the police. I want to make that clear." Jacob knew better than to dissuade anyone from contacting authorities if they saw a need.

"I'm good. Need me to come with you?"

"Nah. I'm taking Throckmorton and a kid from the lab, and until we know more, we need to limit our contact with people as much as possible. We're wearing masks, of course. I'll be in touch."

Jacob called Barbara's number with no success. He called Throckmorton and Khola at the lab and told them he would pick both up, and drive to Mrs. Harvey's house. When they turned onto her street, Jacob's pulse quickened as he noticed smoke rising from a spot a few blocks up. As they drew nearer, he knew whose house was responsible for the faint but obvious gray smoke wafting from the house like his uncle Darrell's pipe smoke on a frigid December day in Michigan. They pulled up to 409 Balboa Street to observe a mound of ashes and brick. Turkey vultures scavenged the exposed refuse, oblivious to or unaffected by the overheated environment beneath them. Large pools of water telegraphed the fire department had come and gone, but they could not have missed the event by more than a few hours.

"God, I hope she wasn't home." He opened the car door and told the others to remain while he searched for any signs of a plant. He spent several minutes combing the disaster and saw no evidence of any plant, much less one Barbara described that night at the YMCA.

Rather than phoning the police to ask if there had been a fatality, when he returned to the car and headed back to the *Arizona Times Herald's* offices, he instructed Khola to comb the internet on his cell phone to see if any fatalities had been reported from the fire. Khola's great grandfather was Norwegian, and his father's name was Nicholas. Khola's mother discovered Kola was the name they used for Nicholas in Norway, so she named their new son Kola. When he was ten years old, he asked his parents if he could add an "h" to his name, and being self-proclaimed hippies from Mount Shasta, California, they agreed.

"I'm going to need you both to spend a little time with me at the office. We need to go over some things and map out a plan. This is not a dead end by any means. Don't worry, we'll compensate you for your time."

When the threesome stepped onto the sixth floor from the elevator, Jacob's eyes landed on his assistant, Tom Bowlsby who was walking quickly toward them, waving frantically. His wire-framed glasses struggled to remain in place. "Mr. Potter! So glad you're back."

"Is it Ted?" he asked, as he approached.

"No. Ted's home. Sawyer called Ted's sister and she's taking responsibility for him. He left his phone here, but she said she would be by to pick it up tomorrow."

"Thanks, Tom, but what's going on?" Jacob could sense uneasiness in the large press room.

"The Governor's office called—said they have unilateral authority to shut down businesses who have employees with a confirmed case of InF. They've claimed police power and say this is reserved to states by the tenth amendment. I did some quick research and listen to this." He plucked a notepad out of his pocket.

"In a 1905 ruling, the Supreme Court observed, and I quote, 'Upon the principle of self-defense, of paramount necessity, a community has the right to protect itself against an epidemic of disease which threatens the safety of its members.' The rep from the office went on to say they can threaten non-compliance with arrest if necessary."

"This is bull-crap," Jacob said as he walked toward his office. "The governor doesn't realize we could just as easily operate from our homes. Bad move, Guvnah." Several staff within earshot glanced up, then quickly resumed their work. "Throckmorton and Khola. In my office! Before they start hurling Molotov cocktails through the windows."

Once in his office, he motioned his guests to sit. Situated on the edge of his desk, he peered over their heads into the busy newsroom, half-expecting paratroopers to come crashing through the ceiling with tear gas canisters. "Okay, guys," as he returned his attention to his guests, "you see what we're dealing with. I realize this is not in your wheelhouse, but you have now seen a burned house and a threat to shut us down. There are other events I can't discuss right now but I am surer than ever there's a concerted effort to cover up past sins."

They both nodded without saying a word, but after a period of silence settled among them, Khola asked, "Are we in danger?"

"If you feel you are, I can't ask you to stay. I can't see anyone doing you harm, but I can't guarantee it won't happen either."

Throckmorton spoke up. "Do you plan on evacuating to your homes or waiting here and challenging authority?"

"I'm going to ask Bowlsby to go home, and if they come knocking or flying through the windows, I'll say I never got the message. Besides, the last time I read something from nineteen-oh-five was . . . well, never."

"I'll stay," Khola said hesitantly. Throckmorton nodded to show his agreement. "This place is giving me pimples on my hemorrhoids." Jacob and Throckmorton both eyeballed him. "Don't ask."

Jacob contacted Dr. Hunter and had him fax a list of patients with their phone numbers who were at the YMCA on Wednesday evening. "All right, guys. This job won't be found on any page in your job descriptions, but we need to call everyone on this list and ask if they still own the plant they received in two thousand."

Jacob had already contacted the Bennington Nursery about the plant Dr. Mata gave them weeks before, but they said it had been bought by a young woman who used cash, and the description given by the cashier that day was so nondescript, he was forced to call it a dead end.

"If you come across someone who gave the plant away, get their name and contact information. If they moved, see if they left it or took it with them. All we need is one plant to help Throckmorton do his research."

"Wouldn't hurt to get more than one," said the gray-templed epidemiologist.

"No argument, but if we find one, we're moving on it quickly. Try calling, then text them if they don't answer. We don't have time for emails. Once we get through this list, we start calling from the *Arizona Times Herald's* distribution list."

The list had been kept in notebooks until Jacob took over from his Uncle Sidney in 1983. Within the first week, a team of typists entered every name, address, and phone number into Microsoft Word, which was a new piece of software which threatened to supplant Word Perfect as the best word processing software on the market.

"We have it broken down demographically and I had Karen run a list of fifty to sixty-year-olds. If we get a hit, we pack up and drive out immediately, and tell them to wait for us. I'll pay one thousand dollars for the plant. That should keep them there. Tell them not to answer the door or their phone until they see us pull up in my white Escalade. Any questions?"

As they shook their heads, Jacob gave each of them three sheets of names. "Throckmorton, you take my office. Khola, take my secretary's office. She's off today."

"Does she have InF?" Khola asked.

"No, it was planned, but you can wear a mask if it makes you feel better. I'll sit at Sylvia's desk. It's been cleaned well since her death. Whoever gets the first hit notifies the other two, and don't worry about a risk of infection. We fumigate the office three times a day with a hydrogen peroxide formula, and no one is allowed to come to work with any InF symptoms."

They spent the next few hours calling and texting but turned up no one who could get their hands on a plant. They found many who had died from previously unknown causes, but from the recent mass coverage of the insomnia flu, most now labeled the cause of death among loved ones as InF. The calls beat them down like a 4th grade German teacher berating your accent. They decided at 4:30, their task was futile. The newsroom was coming alive in preparation for the next day's edition, but it would lack any news of a breakthrough. Maybe tomorrow would bring hope.

48

The front page of the *Arizona Times Herald* on July 16 read, "The Gift Which Keeps on Giving? Y2K Plant is Killing Twenty Years Later."

Jacob ran with the story, which lacked a motive, a suspect, and a cure, but it caught the attention of Phoenix, along with cities across the U.S., nonetheless. Calls came into the office non-stop and were a mix of anxiety-ridden readers and fifty-somethings asking if the plant they received would eventually be their death knell.

"We certainly have the city talking," Bowlsby said. "You were right about setting up that separate line and reward for plant owners. So far, thirty-nine plants have been dropped off and more on the way. We have the boys at the lab picking them up in their hazmat gear."

"That's not all," said Jacob. "In the last hour, I've had calls from the CDC, Stanford's epidemiology department, and a conspiracy theorist's group who calls themselves the NIC—Nothing Is Coincidence. I finally put the Do Not Disturb button on my phone so I could get some work done." Jacob's appearance nailed the part of the disheveled, sleepless newspaper guy.

Tom started toward the door, "Oh, I almost forgot." He raised a finger and turned back toward Jacob. "Ted in the mailroom received a plant for his thirty-third birthday. I'm sure you were going to ask about him, but he came up this morning to tell us."

Jacob shook his head slowly.

"What's even more interesting is his older sister lived with them back then, and she died three years ago. The doctors said it was early dementia and encephalitis, but Ted's convinced it was the InF now, and he doesn't want to die like she did."

Jacob attempted to hide a puzzled look. "How many sisters does Ted have?"

"Just the one who died. Why do you ask?"

"No reason. Just curious."

After Tom left his office, Jacob jotted down some notes.

1. Who the heck is Ted's sister? Who picked him up?

2. FBI. Decide if we involve them.

3. Marie. Why has she shut down?

49

The Natives Are Getting Restless

Arizona Times Herald. Editorial reprint from Wisconsin State Journal. July 17, 2021, Milwaukee, Wisconsin.

Just ten days ago, Governor Fortney was quoted as saying, "What we are seeing is a simple variant of the coronavirus." But after his younger sister developed very different symptoms—those attributed to what we now know as the insomnia flu—his opinion has taken a sharp turn. "This is a very different disease. We do not yet know of its reach, we are blinded to the cause, and we are, if you believe the talking heads, light years from a cure, but the CDC continues to be silent with respect to this enemy we now face. We must not allow this new insult to cripple us, and as your governor, I intend to marshal all available resources to bring an end to what I feel is a terrorist attack on the citizenry of Wisconsin." Though Fortney put on a brave face, he is viewed by many as a governor in his final term. His handling of the newest pandemic has been scrutinized relentlessly, and we raise our hands when asked who has piled on. If you are a praying person, we ask for your intercession. If not . . . well, maybe it's time for a conversion.

Jilian confided in Marie as they sat on the edge of a dock on the south side of Kyle's lake, named Lake Veracity after software he created for his profession. They wore shorts and tank tops, borrowed from Kristy, and liberally applied a layer of sunscreen.

"Just got a text from an ex-boyfriend. He's the governor of Wisconsin and he's struggling with this thing. I know it's all over the country, but it may ruin his career. Feel bad for the guy."

"You have all kinds of secrets, girl."

Jilian shook her head slowly. "I'd rather not have any. You know, Dr. Hunter's very kind to let us to stay here, but I can't keep hiding like this."

"I've got patients who need me as well. Telemed works great, but some of my seniors haven't embraced technology, so I need to get back for them. Even though they're likely out of the age range for the new flu, it doesn't make them less anxious."

Jilian tossed some game fish grower to a knot of catfish, who eagerly awaited each meal offering. "Anyone contacted your office about your visit to the hospital?"

"Not so far," said Marie. "I told them to let me know if anyone came by. So far, nothing."

"Maybe we're making a shark out of a guppy. I know I had a guard at my door, but how do we know he was a bad guy?" Jilian hurled more chum into the water. Her ribs ached with each throw, but it was a good ache . . . the kind that gives you options. She could put down the fish food and stop—an avoidance decision, which was a behavior absent from her genes. If she owned that DNA, she would have chucked Senator Bonner's postmortem note and moved back home to Okinawa. The other choice was to face hurdles as a challenge. The pain she felt in her chest would be a reminder someone tried to kill her or did not care if she was killed. This was a memory she wanted to keep fresh. She tossed another handful to the hungry catfish.

Marie stood. "Of course, you're right. We don't know if any-one means us harm, but we still need to be careful. What Kyle told us this morning . . . gunshots at the Y? Too much is happening." She shivered as she thought about the warning from the two on motorcycles. She knew they could not hide. Would she endanger Jilian if she told her about them? She could not and would not take the chance.

A light sprinkle forced them inside, where they saw Kyle at work behind the desk he had built from his grandfather's oak tree. It was the same oak which was split during a 1948 lightning storm in Bertram, Texas that crashed through the kitchen and killed his grandmother—the only girl John Paul Sr. ever dated. Kyle's father was six at the time, his aunt Merene four. His grandfather became bitter. He blamed God, turned away from his Baptist family, and eventually shot his business partner.

Soon after, he swam under Buchanan Dam and tied himself to a pillar. It was a futile attempt to prevent anyone from finding his body. Scuba divers located it after it was reported John Paul Hunter had been seen jumping in the lake on the anniversary of his wife's death. Kyle used the tree as both a memorial to his grandma Matha and as a solemn and unspoken admonition to keep large trees away from his home.

Marie spoke up first. "We're thinking of blowing this joint, Kyle. You've been a great host, but we have to get back to our lives."

"Speak for yourself," Jilian said. "The governor—and I hate calling him that—went through the back door and is trying to get me disbarred over what he calls, 'failure to disclose.' He said I should've alerted the constituency sooner about Senator Bonner's contraction of the insomnia flu. I resigned my position in the senator's office, of course. He used the seventeenth amendment to appoint Bradley to take her place, and the bastard opened an investigation while I was in the hospital." Her neck colored under her Polynesian complexion. "I won't be scared into hiding out here but may stick around to plan the next stage in my life."

"Stay as long as you like," Kyle said.

"Thank you. I won't take advantage of you, but the view here . . . the tranquility . . . it's hard to leave."

50

"We have some news," said Throckmorton.

Jacob had been sitting at his desk for hours, getting very little work done, as he waited for the lab. "Thanks for calling. What've you got?"

"I could have called an hour ago, but we wanted to make sure."

"And?"

"You won't like it. We found no evidence of prions in any of the plants."

Jacob sat with the phone pressed to his ear, stunned at what he just heard. "That doesn't make sense. We were so sure. Can you run the tests again? Any way you could have missed something?"

"Let's put it this way. I'm not saying there was *never* any presence of prions on the plants. All I'm saying is there is no trace now. If there were, they've magically disappeared."

"What about fingerprints?" Jacob's knowledge of forensics was limited to a few episodes of *Murder She Wrote*. "Did the guys get any that were common to more than one pot?"

"Again, no good news there. I guess twenty years on ceramic

does a number on *any* prints. For all we know, the distribution company was ordered to have their delivery guys use gloves. It wouldn't surprise me if they thought that far ahead."

Jacob thought for a minute as he left Throckmorton hanging. "I've got a call to make. Let me know if you turn up anything." He ended the call, pulled Ted's phone out of his desk drawer, and punched in a number found in recent calls. There was no answer, so he left a voice mail. "I've got more questions. Let me know when and where we can meet."

He then used his own phone to call Marie, who answered distressfully on the third ring.

"Hey. Sorry. Just getting in the car."

"Where you going?"

"I can't stay hidden forever." She put him on speaker, started her car and backed it slowly out of Kyle's long and winding driveway.

"I'm worried about you," said Jacob. "We don't know who's behind the explosion, and now I've gotten you involved. I'm so sorry."

"Don't see you had much choice. Jilian might not be alive right now if we hadn't intervened." She punched in her office address to the GPS system.

"That doesn't make me feel any better, but I see you're equally concerned about the situation. Why don't you—"

"Jacob, I'm sorry, but I have to go." She terminated the call, bit her lower lip, and drove toward town.

Jacob stared at his phone and wondered again what was going on with Marie. Ted's phone chirped. "Luca! Thanks for calling back." There was no response. Jacob could hear road noise on the other end. "Who is this?" After a few seconds, the connection ended.

51

Sawyer loaded his two boys into the Jeep Wrangler and headed to his sister's house on the other side of Scottsdale. His sons had not seen their mother in more than two years. When he told her story, few believed. His Victoria ran off with the circus which came to town in the summer of 2019. An affair with the ringmaster notwithstanding, she had always dreamed of such an odyssey. She watched *The Greatest Showman* over one hundred times, and when her lithium ran out that weekend, she left without packing. Her billfold, driver's license, and passport still occupied the dresser drawer at 7165 Oak Lane, Scottsdale, Arizona. Sawyer would open the drawer sometimes, hoping she had returned and retrieved her things, but his checks became less frequent over the last two years.

When he arrived, his sister waited at the door. "Before you say anything, it's no trouble. I know you wouldn't leave them if it wasn't important."

"Thanks, Bailey. It won't be for more than a few days."

"It's all right. Come on in, boys," she said as she waved them inside the three-story Victorian home their parents left them after their death in the Pentagon on September 11, 2001. "Let's see if there's any ice cream in the freezer."

Sawyer smiled, shook his head, climbed back into the jeep, and drove away. Bailey took the boys to the kitchen where a large overalled man with thinning white hair enjoyed a sandwich. "Ted, meet Derrall and Weldon. Boys, meet Mr. Ted."

52

Jacob drove his Escalade out of the parking garage and onto Fitzhugh. He took a right at the light onto seventh and headed north. He welcomed the cloudy day with a late afternoon sprinkle, which activated his wipers. As he reached for the volume button to see if KTAR was reporting any breaking news, his peripheral vision caught frantic movement through the window of a Range Rover Sport on his right. He recognized Luca waving, then motioning him to follow. Jacob nodded, then followed him down seventh, and turned onto Montford. A few blocks later, Luca turned into the Cunningham mall lot and parked under a tree at the empty northeast corner. Jacob eased up beside him as Luca stepped out. He waved him over to a curb under the tree.

"What's this all about, Luca?" The sprinkle abated somewhat, but with the shield of the desert willow above them, Jacob was not sure. Determined shoppers entered and exited the mall doors, taking advantage of an industry which had been near imploding during the recent pandemic. Highway patrolmen were busy in the distance as the Loop had been snarled with a wreck. Jacob assumed the slick overpass was to blame.

Luca uneasily surveyed those surroundings, then turned to Jacob. "Did you happen to receive a call on Ted's phone from my phone lately?"

"Yes. I left you a message, and someone called the phone, but said nothing. Who was that?"

Luca hung his head and slowly shook it. "I don't know, but that was a test to see if anyone was following me. Sorry I didn't warn you."

His new friend appeared stressed. He had not shaved in days, his shoulders slumped, and Jacob noticed a head-tilt tic he had not noticed before. "I've got some questions for you, but first, tell me what's going on." Jacob placed his hand on Luca's shoulder and squeezed. "I'll do anything I can to help."

Luca nodded. "Thanks. Let me back up a few days. I never told you about Artimus, but he was another friend of mine and Enzo's. We confided in him after our discovery in 1999 because he had completed some seminal research into prion transmissions. He was very helpful but kept his distance. Wanted his name kept out of every reference. He was never clear about his reasons for the distrust, but we never probed too deeply. He was too valuable to compromise our relationship."

"So, that's why you haven't mentioned him before now? What changed?" The rain intensified and the willow above them slowly began to surrender to the skies.

"His wife, April, called me on Tuesday. She'd been out of the country for two weeks visiting her parents in Milan. When she came home, she found him hanging in their garage. It appeared to be suicide, but she insisted it wasn't."

Jacob flinched. "Did she contact the police?"

"Of course. It was ruled a suicide, but April doesn't believe it."

Luca nodded in agreement. "She said he had just bought a new boat and was excited about taking her out on the lake."

"Where was this?" Jacob assumed it was not local, or his paper would have covered it.

"They live . . . or did live . . . in Utah.

"So, what about the phone?"

"After April's call, I panicked," Luca said. "It felt like someone was watching me. When I would drive, I could feel cars tailing me. I couldn't think straight. Thought about flying back home, but now with two friends dead . . . it didn't feel right."

"I'm glad you stayed," said Jacob. "Thank you."

"I grew eyes in the back of my head in my twenties. They keep me on edge."

Jacob was worried about his new friend's mental state. A neurotic bent could lead to a lack of focus. "So . . . the phone?"

"I pulled into a truck stop a few days ago. Found a door of an eighteen-wheeler with a New Mexico license plate unlocked and stuffed the phone under some paperwork in the glove compartment. Then I abandoned my rental car in a parking garage and bought this used jeep from a personal ad in your paper."

Jacob eyed Luca as raindrops continued to wet their faces. "Trying to grow a beard as well?"

"Yes. And I'll be dying my hair black this evening."

"Sounds like you've thought of everything."

Luca shook his head. "No, I'll never think of everything. I'm just doing what I can to stay alive and find out what happened to my friends."

"So, the phone call—"

"If I were you, I'd get rid of that phone."

Jacob thought of Ted's phone in the desk drawer of his office. "Let me make a call."

Luca nodded.

Jacob scrolled until he found the number and punched it. "What's up?"

"Tom, are you still at the office?"

"Just left. Need me to go back?"

"Yes. I need you to get the phone out of my desk drawer. It's in the one on the bottom behind the files. I need you to package it up, put an address on it I will text to you, then take it to the post office on Lexington and drop it in the overnight chute. Have you got that?"

"Yes sir. On it. Let you know if I hit any snags."

"Thanks." Jacob ended the call and texted him the address. "Now let's talk prions."

"What would you like to know?" asked Luca.

"This may take a while, and I'll need to take some good notes, so can we navigate to a dryer place? There's a bar across the highway called Dave's that Tom told me about. I've never been there, so hopefully we won't draw any attention. Follow me there?"

"Sure."

Dave's bar would generously be described as eclectic. A Pabst Blue Ribbon neon sign flickered above the aged and gold-specked mirror behind the bar. A gentleman with dark blue coveralls swayed in a stool at the north end. The hand he waved erratically was ignored by the bartender. Cigar smoke replaced a considerable percentage of the oxygen, but Jacob could not see a single smoker in the house. He thought the owner must pump it in for atmosphere. A band of misfit musicians was in the process of tuning their instruments on a stage which covered fewer square feet than a coffee table.

After they found seats in a booth and ordered drinks from a septuagenarian who could have been attractive in a 1972 dimly lit nightclub after four Long Island iced teas, Jacob asked Luca, "So, Throckmorton had several—"

"WhoWho is this Throckmorton?"

"Sorry. Getting ahead of myself. He's my epidemiologist contact."

"Can he be trusted?" Luca spoke in a whisper, although the tinny cover band made an effort to entertain customers of the Holiday Inn three blocks away.

"I checked his background and feel very good about him."

Luca took a long gulp of his beer, wiped his mouth, and nodded. "I hope you're right. I have a hard time trusting anyone right now."

Jacob struggled to hear him over the noise but read his lips with the help of the illuminated digital table menu, which fit this establishment like a sumo wrestler playing the harp. "So, Throckmorton said he and his lab guys checked more than forty plants we know were delivered by this Brand New Horizons company, and there was not a single trace of prions on any of them."

Luca shook his head before Jacob finished his revelation. "Of course not! After twenty years of watering, transpiration, the exchange of oxygen and carbon dioxide and trimming of branches and leaves, this doesn't surprise me at all. Hell, it's not even the same plant anymore after so many years."

Jacob felt both ignorant and defeated. "I guess the prions could also have died by now from air fresheners—maybe extreme temperatures, and just the passage of time as well."

"Oh no," Luca responded. "Prions are not that easily killed. They resist almost every method of destruction—fire, ionizing radiation, disinfectants—even autoclaving can't destroy them."

"Knowing this, is there any chance at all a prion could have hung around any of the plants after twenty years?"

"Theoretically, no. I don't know what type of miracle it would take, but if I were you, I'd climb another tree."

53

Sawyer called in sick. 102 temp. Will report back
when feeling better.

The text from Tom Bowlsby did not make sense to Kira after
their ride yesterday when he had an abundance of energy. *Must
be something he ate.* Anytime they were together, and it was time
for lunch, he would suggest anything from Ethiopian cuisine to
Mongolian stir fries. She would rather have a buffet selection from
Souper Salad. She decided to drive to his home in Scottsdale to see
if there was anything she could do for him. Fifteen minutes later,
as she drove onto Oak Lane, she saw his jeep at the end of the street
driving away from his French Country styled home. Thinking
anyone with a temperature over one hundred should not be out
driving, she followed him, using skills she learned at the police
academy—skills she never used, after her father's death in a drug
bust elbowed her away from the police force and into journalism.

As he headed out of Scottsdale, she checked her charge, and
worried this might be a longer trip than she had planned.

He headed south, and after he entered Chandler, he turned on Crescent, then took a right onto Dempsey. When he slowed, it appeared to Kira he was searching for an address. She pulled into an empty driveway and hoped the owner was away. She turned on her cell phone camera and began taking photos.

Sawyer parked on the side of the street she was on, then walked back down the sidewalk toward her. He carried a dark blue duffle bag and consistently angled his head left. She quickly ducked down below her window, thankful a hedge of pampas grass would serve to obscure his line of sight to her Tesla. He was four houses away when she used her remote-control lever for the left side driver's mirror and swiveled it to allow her a view down the sidewalk. Just as she angled it enough to see him, he darted between two houses and disappeared. She debated whether to get out and follow him, but seeing another row of houses behind this one, separated by an alley, he was likely going to enter one of the two on this side. She chose to remain crouched low in her seat, vigilantly eyeing the rotated mirror.

She only had to wait a few minutes before he reappeared. She watched him plunk the duffle bag into his trunk, then quickly get in and drive off. Kira hastily backed out of the driveway, and as she followed Sawyer again, she took some quick photos of the two homes, ensuring the addresses on the mailboxes were in the photos. 1436 and 1438 Dempsey. She continued to follow at a distance as he merged onto I 10 headed to Sky Harbor Airport.

When he neared the exit, and it became clear where he was going, her mind raced. She wondered about a lover out of town, but with a wife who ran away with the circus two years ago, who could blame him? Maybe he had a gambling addiction and was headed to Vegas. After all, he did live large, even before Catherine left. Perhaps he just needed to get away. With the death of Danny, maybe he needed some time to decompress. Her curiosity was piqued further when she saw him park his car in the long-term lot and take a tram to Terminal 4. She followed the tram, parked on the curb, and followed him inside.

She noticed his bag was no longer the blue duffle he had taken between the two houses, but a large black bag he would need to check. When she saw him get in an American Airlines line, she counted twelve passengers ahead of him. She quickly located a Drugs and More shop and purchased a large yellow suitcase on rollers, a gray toboggan, a neck pillow, and the largest pair of sunglasses in the store. She went to the line Sawyer was in and inserted herself with two people between them.

She pulled up her American Airlines app while she watched Sawyer in her periphery and found three flights leaving in the next hour. One to Dallas, one to Chicago and one to Milan, Italy. After he checked his bag and walked toward the gate, she waited her turn, then let the pregnant blonde go in front of her so she could get the same reservationist Sawyer had. She hurried up to the auburn-haired ticket agent and breathlessly blurted, "That man you just checked in with the brown hair and blue denim shirt—"

"Ma'am, I need your ticket and ID, please."

"I know, but I'm freaking out because that man is my ex-husband, and I have a restraining order against him. I'm flying to Dallas, and I'm not supposed to be on the same plane with him. Court orders. If I—"

"Miss," the agent interrupted, "he's going to Milan, so you have no worries. Perhaps you can wait before entering the security line. You have some time. Now may I see your ticket and ID? Will you be checking the one bag to Dallas?"

Kira slapped her hand over her mouth, contorted her face into a stressed caricature, and moistened her eyes like a seasoned actor. "I can't believe this! I left my billfold in the car! I'll be right back!"

As she ran toward the exit door, the yellow roller bag bounced off a waiting line stanchion and toppled it. She heard the redhead yell, "Better hurry! Bags have to be checked in ten minutes for your flight!"

Once back in her car, just in time to prevent a young airport policeman from placing a TOW sticker under her windshield wiper, she threw the suitcase into the back seat, caught her breath, allowed her pulse to slow and pulled away from the airport. She tossed the toboggan and neck pillow into the seat beside her. *Milan, Italy?* Now that she had collected some intel on her coworker, what would she do with it? Tell Tom, who had called her about his being sick? Jacob? No, this was none of her business. Sawyer could go anywhere he wanted. She had work to do, and she had already wasted enough time following him.

54

Marie drove the twenty-five miles to her office from Kyle's lake house and checked her rearview mirror every few seconds for any motorcycles in pursuit. She was relieved to see none, though her tension as she gripped the steering wheel left her with aching arms as she pulled into the four-story parking garage. She chose a spot with a good view of her office window. She knew she would feel better if she could see her Prius through the blinds. When a bicycle was not her mode of transportation, she preferred a car with the best gas mileage—something ingrained since her childhood when her father ventilated with regularity the virtues of frugality.

Inside her office, she changed into a new dress from her closet, touched up her makeup and slid into a clean, ankle-length clinic jacket. Like Roosevelt Dam stops water from entering Roosevelt Lake, she learned early in her career to leave her emotional baggage at the door. Her life away from the office was not allowed to follow her through the employee entrance. It would prove to be a struggle today, but she listened intently to patients as they revealed symptoms which gave her an indication of their spot on the terminal insomnia flu timeline.

As she counselled a couple in exam room number three, two bull-necked men in dark suits entered the reception area and walked to the front desk. They each held up ID cards and told Rosalinda they were with the FBI and would like to speak with Dr. Jimmerson. While the young receptionist accepted the cards and considered her next action, Marie walked back to her private office to eat a quick protein bar. She rarely took a lunch break, but today, her assistant Uthra told her she had enough time to throw down a quick snack before the next patient required her attention. When she opened the door, Jacob stood up from her chair and put his finger over his lips.

"What are you doing here?" Marie asked in a breathy whisper.

"We don't have much time," he said quickly. "I called your office and they told me you were coming in to see patients, so I drove over and didn't like what I saw."

"Would you please—"

"Let me finish. When I drove up, I saw two men get out of an unmarked car and walk toward your front door. I called your office back and talked to Rosalinda. I told her to text me with how they represented themselves. Don't have time to show you that text, but they claimed to be with the FBI. I called my contact there and they haven't sent anyone to your office. We need to get out of here fast."

Marie had already removed her jacket and grabbed her purse. "How'd you get in here?"

"One of your employees was leaving for lunch, I guess. I slipped through the back door, and she was so engrossed with a phone call—she didn't even pay attention to me." They were out her door and hurried down the hall now.

"Remind me to have a security team meeting when this is over."

Jacob opened the employee door enough to see no one outside who appeared suspicious. He reached into the inside pocket of his sport coat, retrieved a Ruger LC9s and handed it to Marie. "Take it." She hesitated, then grabbed it and dropped it in her purse. "Let's take my car." She followed him to his Escalade and climbed in the passenger seat. As they left the parking lot, the two men burst through the employee door and ran toward their own black Audi S4.

Jacob wished he had disabled it earlier, but no time to lament missed opportunities. He could see one of them in the rear-view mirror pointing their way, so he picked up speed and headed down Cypress.

"Just got a text from Rosie," Marie said. "She says they forced their way through the office to get to the back and when Elizabeth tried to stop them, they shot her. Said they called 911. Don't know more details, but this is scary. God, Jacob, what have we gotten involved with?"

Jacob shook his head as he turned and sped along Seventh. A hundred yards behind them, the Audi screeched around the corner and continued the pursuit. As a former reporter who had traveled every area of Phoenix, he felt like he knew the area better than whoever was behind them, but if they had attempted to kill already, they would stop at nothing. He considered heading toward the police station but thought the two men might be duplicitous officers who could sense the direction and call ahead to arrange an interruption in their flight for safety.

Jacob took a quick left onto Pendleton and handed his cell to Marie. "Look up Ford in my contacts and call the number for me." He ran through stop signs and red lights, and narrowly avoided several accidents. He irritated enough drivers to start a symphony of horns. The Audi gained on them until he saw it collide with a

UPS truck and spin ninety degrees. When he thought their attention was diverted, he turned onto Eleventh.

Marie handed him the phone. "It's Jason."

"Hey J. I need to bring in the Escalade. Can I come right
now?" He took another right.

"Jacob, we're a bit backed up, so—"

"Bringing it in now!" He disconnected and handed it back to
Marie. "In case he calls back." He sped through a few more stop
signs and entered I17. He edged the speedometer to ninety, then
glanced in the mirror and saw no sign of the Audi. He exited onto
Throckmorton, crossed under the highway at the light and drove
five miles north to Dunwoody Ford. He pulled into the service
bay and jumped out. Marie followed.

Jason met them and before he could say anything, Jacob
tossed him the key and said, "Needs a tune up and a new passenger mirror." The car's appendage had been shorn off on a close
encounter with a stop sign. "We're going inside to get a rental.
This is Dr. Jimmerson, and she's got a flight to catch in forty-five
minutes. Can we make this quick?"

"Sure thing, Jacob. We can—"

Jacob and Marie had already rushed through the service door
and were headed to the counter. "We need the fastest Mustang
you have."

The green-haired girl with a Santa Claus build finished
thumbing a text, carefully avoiding her three-inch striped fingernails, then regarded him indifferently. "That would be the
Mach-E, but there's an extra charge for—"

"I don't care," Jacob said emphatically. "You have my credit
card on file. Potter, Jacob Potter. We have a flight to catch. Can
you point me to the Mach-E and get me the key quickly?"

"Why, yes, Mr. Potter. I'll call them right now to let them

know you're on your way." She pointed to a door on her left. "It's right through that—"

They were through before she could finish. As they hurriedly found seats in the leather interior, Jacob asked the service tech who gave him the keys, "Is there an exit through your used car lot in back?"

"Mr. Potter, we need to do an inspection of any scrapes and dents—"

"No time. I'm sure it's fine. Exit?"

"Yes, you'll see it once you get past the line of Explorers. It dumps you onto Anthem."

"Thanks." They took off, found the exit, then headed down the street named after an insurance company. "Best if you lie down in the seat. They're searching for two people." Marie laid her head on the console. Jacob was thankful she was small enough to exercise this move with little trouble.

He angled back onto I17 and headed north. When he saw a Holiday Inn Express, he exited and turned right off the access road into the front drive. "Don't get up yet." He got out and pretended to stretch, as if he had been driving for hours. He scanned the area, and when he saw nothing unusual in the surroundings—and no black Audi—he ducked his head back in the car. "It's clear."

As they walked toward the revolving door, Jacob plugged in the gait song "Hotel California" to his mental CD player. He changed the words to "Hotel Arizona" and smiled as he walked in sync to the beat. As they arrived at the registration desk, an attractive, olive-skinned girl with a Manuela nametag acknowledged them over reading glasses with a broad smile. "Welcome to the Holiday Inn! Checking in?" The thick Columbian accent added some charm to the greeting.

Jacob pulled out his billfold and passed an Amex card across the desk, then sneered at the atomic clock on the wall behind the young lady. "I'm a private investigator and have just extricated Mrs. Jones from a critical situation. I can only say her husband's been stalking her and is threatening to kill her. There is no reason to think he will show up here, but I need you to put her up in a room with a window at the end of the hall which has a view of your front door. She will also need some toiletries. Had to make a quick exit from a very volatile environment. I'm sure you understand."

"Of course, sir. You didn't have any chance to pack a suitcase at all, did you sweetie?"

"I'm afraid not," said Marie, looking the part of an abused spouse.

"I'll be back with some clothes for her," said Jacob. "I can't emphasize enough how important it is you keep her presence here secret. Her ex is quite wealthy. One of those guys who runs a corporate Medicaid mill. He's made millions on the backs of the poor and the government teat and he'll stop at nothing to find her. We know he's got two of his men out searching. If you see a black Audi with two guys who lost their necks, please text me at this number." He slid a card across the desk after writing his number on the back.

"This says you're with the *Arizona Times Herald*," she said.

"That's right. They contract my services and want me to use their cards. It's all about publicity these days, and you know the saying: 'There's no such thing as bad publicity.' I'll be back in an hour. Please take care of her, Manuela. I owe ya."

"I certainly will." She ran his card, then handed it back to Jacob, who pocketed it and quickly left.

"Come this way, Ms. . . . Jones. I'll show you to your room."

55

After Marie left Kyle's lake house, Jilian decided to hang back and enjoy the peace and quiet. She turned off her cell phone to augment the effort. The incessant spam calls and texts kept her on edge, but not today. Nope. Not today. She could get plenty of work done here on her laptop, and truthfully, she felt better about having Kyle around to change her dressings and help her heal faster. The effects of the explosion were still fresh, both mentally and physically, so even though being forced into seclusion gnawed at her moxie, she was in no rush to head back into the maelstrom of city life. She sat on a porch swing in the back yard and worked through some loose ends for the late Senator Bonner. Kyle walked through the back door.

"You and the senator were very close. I admired her tenacity and transparency. Do you deserve much of that credit?"

"Not at all. She was the real thing. Arizona lost a diamond when she passed." Jilian Quito waxed melancholy anytime she thought about the character of her good friend. The sun ducked behind a dark gray cloud, and a cool breeze off the lake wafted in an array of pleasant scents. Freshly mowed grass, cherry laurels and black cherry contributed to a coalescence of smells Kyle called a "symphony of scents."

"Tell me more about her," he said as he sat on the other end of the swing. "Something us commoners would've never known."

Jilian closed her laptop and laid it beside her on the swing. "She was very private, of course. Never got elected for her bombasity, but that's no secret. I was a confidante, so she shared more with me than I would be willing to detail, but one thing many never knew was how good she was at playing pool."

"True," said Kyle. "Never heard that."

"In fact, she paid her way through college by beating guys who fancied themselves to be pool sharks. They had no idea they were being sharked. One idiot bet his car—and lost." She laughed. "It was an old Toyota Celica, but it was his only ride."

Kyle smiled. "I bet pool sharks make good politicians."

"It didn't hurt her. She could always play that game."

"What else?" Kyle asked. "What was her favorite food?"

"Oh, that's easy. Krispy Kreme donuts. She could afford to eat them because she ran five miles every day, but if she didn't run, she could've ballooned up to a few hundred pounds. She used to knock on my office door at the end of a day. When I opened it to find her wearing running shorts, she would hold up a donut." Jilian held her arm up high. "She'd say, 'Going for a Krispy run. You in?' You can tell by my shape, I never joined her."

Kyle smiled. "Do you think you can have any influence on carrying on those projects she was heavily invested in?"

"I doubt it, but that won't stop me from trying. They're jockeying to get me disbarred, but they don't have a case, and even if they did, I can work some magic." Before joining the senator's team, Jilian had won her last twenty-three jury trials.

Kyle was not surprised. He was content to have her on his side, though he was not sure how many sides there were. "You mentioned Kevin Sandam getting close to the governor."

"Yes?"

"I've been thinking about that ever since you mentioned him. It bothered me until I researched my father's patient files and found him. But the oddest thing—and I think that's why I remembered his name. I recall my dad talking about the guy who changed his name completely. It wasn't unusual to change a first or last name, but both? From his chart, he changed it in 1996. No notes about why. I suppose that was too personal to put in his file, and Dad never mentioned it if he knew. I guess with Sandam's death, we may never know."

Jilian thought about what Kyle said. "I'm not sure that's important, but I agree changing both names is rare."

"Maybe he just didn't like his name? It didn't sound offensive to me. He was Alex Bergfield before."

"Maybe it wasn't that he disliked his original name. Perhaps he did it to honor someone."

"I considered that," said Kyle, "but I found no other Sandams that would trigger that. No, the only reason that makes sense is he did it to hide, but from whom?"

"Again, we may never know, and I'm not sure these mental gymnastics are worth the effort."

"I'm sure you're right, I'm sure you're right."

56

After Kira parked her car and plugged it into the Tesla charger, she removed her laptop from her backpack and set it on her desk. When it booted up, she did an address search for 1436 and 1438 Dempsey. After several minutes of searching for the owners of the two homes she watched Sawyer maneuver between, she called Taylor at the *Arizona Times Herald*.

"This is Taylor."

"Thanks for answering, girl. Need a favor."

"Shoot. Anything for you."

"Need you to utilize our internal database and tell me the residents of 1436 Dempsey and 1438 Dempsey."

"Hold on."

Kira heard the keystrokes over the connection.

"Got it. 1436 belongs to a Kylie Houston and 1438 has a Jilian Quito registered as the owner."

Kira sat stunned, as she heard what she hoped she would not. "I've gotta go," she eventually managed to say. "Thanks." She ended the call, then punched in Jilian's number. It rang three times, then went to voicemail.

"You've reached Jilian. If this is a real person, feel free to leave a message and I'll return the call as soon as possible. Have a blessed day." *Beep*!

"Jilian, this is Kira. Please call me back! You may be in danger. Do *not* go to your house!" She ended the connection, then decided to drive to Kyle's lake house. She hoped she was still there. As she merged onto I 10, she tried Kyle's phone, but after a few rings, she saw a call coming in from the *Arizona Times Herald* and took that call instead.

"This is Kira."

"There's been an explosion in Chandler. You're the closest, so Tom wants you there ASAP."

"What's the address?" Kira's hand shook uncontrollably, making it difficult to hold her phone.

"We don't have it yet. We received a call from a citizen a few blocks away. He was out mowing his lawn and said the sound was so disturbing he almost ran over his dog with the mower. Said he saw smoke rising, and flames were starting to appear. Sounds like you can locate it easily once you get into Chandler."

Kira mindlessly ended the call, then mustered enough strength to punch in 1438 Dempsey to her GPS and began the eight-minute drive. She struggled to concentrate on her destination as visions of her coworker planting a bomb pummeled her thoughts. She wanted to think the best of Sawyer, but it proved difficult after observing his behavior. Even before she entered Chandler, she could see smoke in the distance. *Maybe she wasn't home*, she thought. Then she prayed she was not.

She turned onto Crescent and glanced down Dempsey Street. The smoke was over several houses now, as wind had picked up and was not consistent in which direction it wanted to blow. She turned on Dempsey and headed toward Jilian's address. When she could see the house, it appeared intact from the front. She parked her car and took the same route Sawyer had taken between the two homes. She felt better when she saw the explosion had occurred in a house on the other side of the alley. It wasn't Jilian's house.

Remembering her assignment, she found the fire truck and police detail in front of the demolished house and approached a uniformed, clean-shaven man with an unlit cigar dangling from the corner of his mouth. As she approached, he pulled the cigar from his mouth and used it as a pointer.

"Ma'am, you'll have to exit this area and stand behind the ropes like the rest of the neighborhood." He pointed the cigar behind him as he finished his admonition.

He had accurately described the gathering behind him as a neighborhood. People were stacked ten-deep behind a row of saw-horses the police had lined up as a perimeter. The two homes on either side of the destroyed home were severely damaged. Other homes nearby had windows which shattered from the explosion and pieces of roof were embedded in the yards across the street. White insulation blanketed cars, homes, and sidewalks nearby.

She pulled a card from her pocket and handed it to the stolid but perspiring Officer Scalene. "I'm with the *Arizona Times Herald*. Are you the officer most capable of answering a few questions?" Kira loved that opening question, as it caught people off guard. Not Scalene. A crew from the Bureau of Alcohol, Tobacco and Firearms had just left after their explosive detecting K9 ruled out any other danger. The fire marshal had also left, leaving Scalene to finish things up.

"No press, ma'am. The FBI's been called in, and I have no comment." He turned away from her to address another offi-cer nearby.

"So, do I write the Phoenix PD was uncooperative in supplying any details—even what *caused* the explosion?"

"You can print this, Ms. Mackin. It's too early to know the cause or whether it was accidental or intentional. If we possessed further information, we would be forthcoming. Now if you'll excuse me—"

"Was anyone inside?" she pushed.

"The only habitant was taken to the hospital. You'll have to check with them to check her status."

"So, it was a woman."

"That's what I was told." Scalene briskly walked away without another word.

Kira knew she could get the name from her database, so she turned toward the destroyed home and shook her head. *This was no accident.*

57

Jacob had just finished buying some clothes for Marie at Desert Sky Mall and stepped into his car when his phone buzzed.

"Luca, what's up?"

"I have some more information to share with you."

"What did you find out?"

"It's not so much what I found out, but information from twenty years ago I haven't shared with you yet."

"Okay." Jacob was not sure how to respond to this.

"We can't do this by phone. When can we meet?"

Jacob started his car and headed toward the Holiday Inn Express. "I've got an errand to run first. Can we meet in an hour?"

"One hour at Dr. Stacey Layman's office. I talked to her office manager, Lesia. She said we could use their conference room. They're about to close right now, but she'll let us in."

"You don't even live here, Luca. How do you already know a doctor?"

"Long story I don't have time for, but I rescued one of her goats. She thanked me by saying she owed me and to let her know if I needed anything while I was in Phoenix. She gave me her card, and I figured that would be a safe place to meet, so I'm calling in the debt."

"Gotta hand it to you, you're resourceful. See you in an hour." Jacob closed the connection, then called Marie as he headed toward the hotel. "Headed your way. Any sign of trouble?"

"Only that they didn't have room service. Considered using my Ruger to force the issue but decided that wasn't wise."

"I can pick up Chinese. Sound good?"

"Perfect." Marie realized she had not eaten all day.

"And you haven't contacted anyone, right?"

"I can follow orders, and yes, I let two calls go to voice mail, so not answering anyone but you."

"See you in ten. Bye."

After he dropped off food and clothes for Marie, cautioning her again to stay in her room but to keep an eye on the front drive through her window, he headed for Knudson Drive to meet Luca. Lesia met him at the front door.

"Dr. Layman had to leave early. One of her goats got out."

Jacob smiled. "I heard about that problem. Luca pulled up just as he started through the door. Jacob waved him in.

Which one of you is Luca?" Lesia asked. Luca raised his hand. "Dr. Layman wanted to thank you again for rescuing Ronald."

"The goat's name was Ronald?"

"Her sense of humor is . . . I'd like to say eclectic, but really it's just corny. She considers Ronald Reagan to be the greatest president ever, so since he's the GOAT, in *her* opinion," she rolled her eyes to reveal her thoughts on the subject, "she named that goat Ronald."

Luca wrinkled his brows. "Why did she call Ronald Reagan a goat?"

"I'll handle this, Lesia. Luca, anytime we think someone is the greatest of all time in their field, usually in sports, we shorten it to GOAT. Greatest of all time. GOAT. Make sense?"

"Ah, now I see. We do not have that acronym in Italy. The way we say the greatest of all time is Il migliore di tutti I tempi, and when I break this down, it's something like 'I'm d tit'."

"Sorry I brought it up," said Lesia. "Let me show you to the consultation room."

They approached the glass enclosure, which had a sign on the door reading, "Without enough sleep, we all become tall two-year-olds."

She waved them in. "There's water in the fridge, but I'm going to the house to make myself a screwdriver. Make yourselves at home. I'll lock up, but you can leave out the back door," she pointed down the hall, "and it will stay locked. Anything else you need?"

"You've been too kind. Please thank Dr. Layman for us," said Jacob.

After the door was closed, Jacob sat in a white leather chair over which he hung his gray sport coat. On the other side of an L-shaped laminated desk, Luca sat in one of two olive-colored chairs and rolled the other out of the way. Jacob chose his position because it gave him a view of the window to his right and the door behind Luca. Recent events had heightened his level of vigilance.

"Appears Dr. Layman is a sleep doctor," said Jacob, referencing the sign on the door and posters in the room, which spoke to the importance of healthy sleep. "Don't you find that coincidental, knowing our concerns about the insomnia flu?"

"I had no idea. Maybe she knows your Dr. Jimmerson. I also had no idea how beautiful the women in your country are."

"We have all types, Luca, but yes, women like Lesia are not hard on the eyes."

"Anyway," continued Luca, "let me start back in college."

Jacob pulled out his pad to take notes. "Sounds like you have some blanks to fill in for me."

Luca smiled. "Yes. Once we discovered how to transmit prions from one species to another using air-borne routes, they began treating us like kings. We were even given luxury homes—"

"Wait. Who treated you this way?"

"We were never told their names. I mean the guys in charge. In fact, we never even met them until they called us into a meeting a few weeks later to discuss our progress on other assignments. They used the code names Poseidon, Falcon and Antioch."

"Once you made the discovery, they believed in you? Gave you more work?"

"Exactly. Now when I say we were treated like royalty, I should also mention we never felt safe. We were given no freedom. We were not allowed to travel and were forced to check in daily. Oh, and we detected some interference on our phones we assumed were recording devices."

"You were in prison."

"It felt like that. By the time they called us into the meeting, our psychosis was profound. We didn't dare tell them about a monoclonal antibody we were close to perfecting. It would prevent abnormal proteins from attaching themselves to normal proteins and spreading. All we needed was to alter the particle size enough to pass through the blood-brain barrier to thwart the prions on the other side."

"English, please."

Luca grinned. "Odd you have to say that to an Italian. All it means is we were close to discovering a cure—not exactly a cure, but a method for stopping the spread of any prion disease. Not just fatal familial insomnia, but any of the variant CJD diseases like BSE—that's Mad Cow, Chronic Wasting Disease, scrapie and even kuru."

Jacob dropped his pen and stared at Luca. "You mean you discovered something like an antidote for prion diseases?"

"Not really an antidote, but the outcome would be the same. Before you ask, we couldn't test it on humans until the first ones became symptomatic—symptoms we knew wouldn't appear for another twenty years. What we didn't anticipate was how ruthless these demi-gods were. They must have assumed we would wait, and when the first news hit of InF affecting people, they put their plan into action. They began removing those of us involved on the research side."

"Did you ever perfect the antibody?"

"We think so, but as long as they held us captive, we couldn't test it on FFI victims or even those who had been infected with BSE. We never told them about our discovery, but after a few years, our lab was mysteriously burned to the ground one night. After that, we managed an escape. It was elaborately planned by Enzo's uncle. We left in the Pizza truck after a delivery, then did a plane, train and automobile journey which, until lately, kept us all safe."

"Were you able to recreate your antibody, and did you perfect it? And when can we get our hands on it?" Jacob was intent on the end game.

"This is where it gets interesting. I've been thinking about the best way to use it for good—and yes, at least we think it's ready for human trial—but also to get revenge for my friends and others who've been killed by these monsters."

"Sounds like you have a plan, but I'm begging you to not allow revenge to delay any plan to save lives."

Luca stood, walked over to the window, and regarded a street with sparse traffic. A seven-story Marriott stood across the street and shielded the office they were in from the scorching afternoon Arizona sun. He scanned the windows on all levels and assessed any potential aberrations. When he was satisfied, he did not sit, but paced as he spoke, his rubber soled Jordans squeaking with each turn.

"When we were invited to this meeting, back in 1998, we were already suspicious. Now keep in mind, we were close to getting the antibody right at this time and were confident we would get there."

Jacob nodded but said nothing.

"We had a plant mailed from a 'Mr. Danino' to the BNH organization, in care of Leticia Tucci. The message read, 'Leticia, I bought this plant in Bali last week and from its history, I feel like it will bring good fortune. Please place in our conference room.'"

"Who was this Mr. Danino?"

"He was the treasurer for BNH, and it was well-known the secretary—Leticia—was enamored with him. What she did *not* know was Danino was gay. Enzo took the opportunity to tell the secretary the day after she had placed the plant in the conference room."

"Go on."

"The plant was one we ordered through the nursery. We didn't impregnate it with prions."

Jacob regarded Luca quizzically. "Then . . . what was the purpose?"

"It was our insurance plan. When we joined them in the meeting and saw the plant was still there, to make sure they remembered it, I commented on how well the plant smelled. Enzo then mentioned his mother owned one and she loved it so much she would talk to it every day—she named it Pietre and always invited friends over to smell it."

"I think I know where this is going," said Jacob.

"Tell me what you're thinking."

"You wanted them to use that type of plant for transmitting prions, but to what end?"

"Two months ago, Enzo mailed a letter to Poseidon, Antioch and Falcon at the BNH headquarters in Padua and labeled it 'For Their Eyes Only,' hoping it would get to them. The message was simple. It said the plant we discussed in 1998 in the conference room—the one we all smelled—had already been doused with the FFI prions. It said if they agreed to send a letter to the *New York Times* which detailed their crimes and explained their complicity, the antibody would be made available to them, after which it would be made available to society."

"That's where it went sideways," Jacob said.

"We expected as much. Or at least I did. I paid to have a new identity created and encouraged Enzo and Artimus to do the same. Their wives wouldn't allow it. They refused to uproot themselves from the comfortable life they had created just because of an invisible threat."

Jacob shook his head in disbelief. "They weren't able to convince them it was a serious situation? Maybe even Enzo and Artimus didn't take the threat seriously."

"Artimus golfed five days a week with college buddies. Just bought a boat for the lake they now live by. His original paranoia must have melted away over time. Enzo had a consulting job with Pfizer that paid him so well he worked when he wanted and kept his wife in Louis Vuitton shoes and Hermes handbags. She wasn't budging."

Jacob considered his own wife. "Women have power over us, my friend, but I am sure you are aware."

"So, apparently, do politicians."

"That's true," Jacob agreed, "but why bring—"

"One of the three who held us captive . . ." Luca hesitated.

"Yes?"

"Was Governor Adair."

"You're sure of this?"

Luca nodded. "It's been over twenty years, but I'm quite sure."

"Do you think you could recognize any of the other two?" Although Jacob was hopeful, he was also circumspect when considering the ramifications.

"Maybe. If they haven't aged much. Adair has beady eyes that remind me of a raven and some moderate kyphosis—"

"Uh—"

"Sorry. It's the scientific name for a hunchback." Luca instinctively arched his back into a stooped position. "He had what we call a Dowager's hump. It can be treated, but it doesn't appear he ever made the effort."

"But they used code names back then."

"Yes. He was the one they called Falcon."

"So, what's *your* real name?" Jacob asked. He had spent a few hours trying to locate any evidence of a Luca from Veneto with a science background but found no one the age of his new friend.

"I'd rather not say. Knowing that could only hurt our odds of surviving this."

"Luca it is. Anything else you can recall about your visits with this Triumvirate?"

"Yes. They sat behind a long rosewood desk. Reminded me of a Supreme Court with only three judges." He chuckled as he realized the contrast. "They always had a carafe of a dark liquor at this desk and after a few visits, we learned they had a taste for cognac. Falcon—now known as Governor Adair, was the provider. They trusted his choices and usually complimented the new label he brought."

Jacob wondered if this trio could have good taste in anything. "What else? They talk about women? Girlfriends? Ever mention another name? Have any distinguishable accents?"

"I'm afraid they were rather tight-lipped about anything other than their liquor. They also wore fedoras and sunglasses and were well-tanned every time we saw them. Like they visited tanning beds daily. They were seated when we entered the room and seated when we left, so all we ever saw were their faces." Luca shivered as he pictured his captors from two decades past.

Jacob nodded, then leaned back in the white chair and swiveled from side to side a few times while he thought, tapping his pen a few times on his lower lip. "That plan you mentioned. The one to get back at your malevolent benefactors. Was that it? Just to make them live in fear?"

Luca shook his head as a smile slowly broke across his face. "Just act one. Now comes the coup de grace."

58

"Judge Stoutmeyer! I'm so glad you called. How can I help you?"

"No, no. I'm calling to offer you *my* help, Jilian."

"Now you've got me curious." Jilian was anxious for more reasons. The judge had never called her. She only had her number in her contacts because Senator Bonner had provided it when she was in the throes of InF.

"But first, I wanted to express my condolences for our good friend's passing. She was not only the finest senator I ever knew, but the finest human."

The judge weighed in at 350 pounds of redheaded German and came with a volume knob set at eighty decibels . . . when she was whispering. No one ever speculated as to her opinion on any topic, which was refreshingly unconventional in a judiciary where opinions were a non sequitur. She was self-made, immigrating from Poland with her blue-collar parents when she was two and learning English before she entered grade school in Rhode Island. She graduated at the top of her class at RWU and after interning under Second Circuit Judge Amalia Kearse, made the move to

Phoenix when George W. Bush appointed her as a district judge. Married and divorced within three years, she doted on her only daughter, Izzy.

"Thank you, Judge. It's so hard to understand why someone that special was taken so quickly." Jilian did her best to maintain composure.

"Speaking of the senator, did she ever mention anything about the Klavian Triumvirate?"

Jilian hesitated, then remembered from Senator Bonner's note the judge had known about the secret group. "Not until after her death."

"She spoke to you from beyond the grave?"

"I wouldn't put it past her. In fact, I'm fairly sure she's been doing that, but no, she left a letter for me to read—"

"Wait. Don't say anything else. This line isn't secure. Can we meet?"

Jilian considered this sudden request, then deflected. "Did you hear about the explosion?"

"Yes, I couldn't believe that. You were the only survivor? Are you doing okay? Where are you?"

Jilian hesitated after hearing this line of questioning. "Yes, just a few scratches. Nothing that won't heal. I'm actually on the move, so I'm not really anywhere. Where do you want to meet?"

"Remember that deli where you, Senator Bonner, and I lunched back in the spring?"

Jilian did recall the lunch and pictured her good friend in better times. "Yes."

"Noon tomorrow?"

"See you then."

Judge Stoutmeyer ended the call, then returned her gaze to her guest.

"You did very well, Judge. That wasn't so hard, was it? Your daughter will live. She'll go to a very nice university out East. She'll probably take after you. She'll make you proud." He raised his gun and fired.

59

Twenty miles away, Jilian hung up, and punched Jacob's number in her "recent" list.

"Potter."

"I need to ask you a question, and I need you to be right."

"I'm doing fine, thanks, Jilian. How are you?"

"I need you to be sure with your answer."

"I'll try, but what's this about?" asked Jacob.

She hesitated. "Who knew I was in the hospital?"

"Hmm. Other than the hospital personnel? And Kira and Marie?"

"Yes."

"Just the oaf in the chair sitting outside your room, and whoever he was working for." Jacob had suspicions.

"And no one else?"

"Nope."

She did not want to say what came next. Senator Bonner and the judge were kindred spirits. They were both divorced, and their daughters roomed together at Creighton. They took vacations together and stayed in the same villa every February in Tulum. This made no sense. "Jacob, I think Judge Stoutmeyer is lying to me. She's even—"

"Wait, wait, wait. What happened?"

Jilian paced rhythmically during the call, but sat now, hoping it would help her better digest the situation. "I don't know. She called me out of the blue. She's never done that. Not in the twelve years we . . . meaning the senator and me . . . not in all the years we've worked together. She's never called me. I don't even know how she got my cell number."

"You're not making any sense. So, she called you—"

"It's not that. She knew about me being in the hospital."

"Well maybe someone—"

"And then she wanted to meet me. She asked about the Triumvirate."

"Why would that have come up?"

"Exactly. The whole call was . . . well, it was off. I mean . . . she didn't sound like the judge I know."

Jacob sensed the chasm between what he knew and reality. "Where were you to meet her?"

"Harriet's Deli. It's the one on—"

"I know the deli." Jacob's sister had worked there when they were in high school.

"She also asked where I was."

"You didn't tell—"

"No. I avoided the question. We're supposed to meet at noon tomorrow."

Jacob slowly thought through a plan. "I know of a hardware store across the street. Down about a block. I'm going to get Tom to meet me there about 11:30 and we'll hang out. I know the owner."

"What should I do?"

"Just stay at Dr. Hunter's. You're still there, right?"

"Yes."

"Tom and I will see if this judge ever shows. I'm familiar with her appearance from some stories we've done on her. She's hard to miss."

The judge spoke four languages fluently until a bullet had silenced her.

60

The next morning, Tom met Jacob at Jerry's Hardware Store. It was 11:35. With Jerry's permission, they picked out two sets of military grade binoculars and stationed themselves at a window through which they could see the entrance to Harriet's Deli. The lunch traffic soon picked up. Cars, taxis, and pedestrians filled the street and sidewalks, creating visual difficulties for the two spotters. They caught glimpses of people entering the deli, but no large redheads.

As soon as the street began to see activity, Tom moved to a window farther down the wall to get a different angle and improve their chances of seeing the Judge. Jacob eyed his watch. *Two minutes to noon. Should be here any minute. Judges are always punctual.*

Deep in thought about the eccentricities of the judicial bench, Jacob jumped, dropping his binoculars when he heard glass shatter and then a loud crash. Stands of flashlights and hunting knives were knocked over, and a set of shelves holding thousands of screws, nuts, bolts, and nails tumbled toward the middle of the store. Then he heard a scream from the cashier.

All of this happened in less than a few seconds. When he focused on the toppled shelving, he found Tom lying beside it. Seeing the shattered window, he fell to the floor and crawled to Tom, who he saw moving as he edged closer. Two more bullets tore through the window in the next seconds, bringing more screams from the woman who was now ducked behind the counter. *He's alive, thank God.* He grabbed his ankle and dragged him toward the interior brick wall underneath the windows.

Tom moaned. Jacob searched for blood but saw nothing other than red welts around his eyes. Fifteen feet away lay a set of shattered binoculars. *They were watching for us. The noonday sun probably bounced off the lenses.* The shooting seemed to have stopped.

Jerry called the police over Jacob's objections. Tom was conscious, sitting up against the wall. He surveyed the damage to his facial bones with his fingers. "It's going to be years before I pick up another set of those, but maybe they saved my life."

"We've gotta get out of here," Jacob said hastily. "Can you crawl? Walk?"

"I'm good."

As they crawled along the wall toward the other side of the store, they saw Jerry and his cashier crouched down behind the counter.

"Jerry, we were never here," Jacob directed, sirens wailing in the distance.

"What? Don't you want to—"

"No, Jerry. I don't have time, but I'll explain later. And don't let Ygrette say anything either. Free ad in next Sunday's paper?"

"You guys were never here," Jerry said, as Ygrette regarded him skeptically.

As they reached the front door, they could see the lights of the police cars up the street.

"Come on," Jacob urged, as he helped Tom stand. They walked quickly to Jacob's Escalade, got in and took off down Butayne Avenue.

"We'll get your car later," said Jacob.

"What if the police—"

"They'll have no reason to investigate your jeep. It's just a vandalism complaint with no victims other than property . . . for now. I know Jerry, and he'd change religions for a free ad in the Sunday *Arizona Times Herald*."

He punched Jilian's number. "Your intuition was spot-on. Remind me not to invite you to our Sunday night poker game. By the way, you're on speaker. Tom's here."

"What happened?" she asked breathlessly.

"Tell you when we see you. But . . . don't think you'll ever see Judge Stoutmeyer again."

"Those bastards."

"Luca and I have a plan," Jacob said. "Stay by your phone. Gotta go." After hanging up, he punched a contact that read "Capri."

"It's been a minute, Jake."

"Got a job. Should just take a few hours. Can you spare the time?"

Tom eyed Jacob quizzically.

The heavily accented voice on the line said, "I have to clean something up. Should be available by two."

"I'll text you the details, C. Appreciate the help."

Capri was Haitian-born and grew up in the streets of a military zone, using a rifle from the age of four. His parents were both killed when he was six, and he attempted to escape to the Unites States in a makeshift raft with another family, but they were caught and taken to Guantanamo Bay. From there, he hid in a barrel of flour bound for Boston and was later taken in by The Home for Little Wanderers. They saw so much promise in the young Capri that a benefactor sent him to the best schools and eventually to law school at Columbia. But his temperament, an amalgamation of mistrust, self-preservation and a logical mind that struggled with the disparity between intellect and the incongruencies of a bastardized society, did not conform to the rules and regulations of jurisprudence. The niche he created involved using a quick negotiating mind with an appreciation for guns and an unshakable and nonrepentant bravado.

61

"Thank you all for coming," Jacob started.

He and Luca decided to bring others into their confidence and fill them in on past and future details. He called Marie to let her know he would be picking her up at the back door of the hotel and texted Kyle, Kira, and Jilian to meet at 8:00 a.m. on the eleventh floor of the Century Building; the offices of the *Arizona Times Herald*. While his new editor put the final touches on the Sunday edition, they sat around the large oak conference table with the door closed and shades drawn. Not taking any chances, Jacob had asked security to run a bug sweep thirty minutes before the meeting.

"I wanted to catch everyone up on what we've learned over the last few days and to give each of you," he scanned the table and caught the eyes of each person "those of you I trust and respect for your specific insight into what we are dealing with, and—aw hell. We need your help. Anything you'd like to say before we lay some heavy stuff on you?"

Marie spoke up first. "You introduced Luca as someone who might have some inside knowledge about the genesis of this new prion disease. And let me say I'm glad to hear you're in agreement this is a prion we're seeing. Mr. Luca, can you tell us more? I think I can speak for the others when I say that is what interests us the most."

Jacob nodded to Luca. He told them of his work with Enzo and Artimus, the three heads of BNH—Poseidon, Antioch, and Falcon, and about the deaths of his two friends.

"Why were you motivated to develop a new transmission vehicle for prions?" asked Kyle.

"We never meant it to be used as an instrument for genocide. Prions fascinated us, and we only wanted to see if it was possible to transmit this way. We knew you could inherit the gene. We learned this from a small area in the Veneto region of Italy."

"That's FFI, right?" asked Marie.

"Correct. We know from the Fore tribe kuru can be transmitted by eating the brains of dead infected victims. We didn't know then, but BSE or Mad Cow prions are passed along the chain in much the same way, but in that situation, it crosses species, and we discovered this was much more difficult."

Jilian spoke up. "Although that's comforting to know, why is it more difficult for prions to cross species?"

"It's all about protein shape," said Luca. "For a misfolded protein—a prion—to influence a healthy protein molecule to fold as well, it needs to sidle up and romance it. If the shapes don't match up, like we see in different species, the relationship is much more difficult to consummate. Not to get crude but imagine how difficult it would be for a male human to have sex with a female elephant. Perhaps not impossible, but very difficult."

"I'm sorry I asked," said Jilian.

Luca smiled. "With the prion manifestation we're now seeing, it's my belief with the high infection rate, we're not dealing with a prion that crossed species. This comes from human tissue. It appears to mimic most closely the FFI disease found in the Italian family. That's fatal familial insomnia, by the way."

"You were right, Marie," Kyle said. Regarding the others, "She came to me early on, saying this resembled, almost mimicked FFI. Only seen in Italy until now."

"It stands to reason," said Luca, "this is coming from the brain tissue of an FFI victim. One difference in FFI is temperatures of victims gyrate from high to low, unlike any other prion disease, and from what we're hearing, the affected in this new infestation are seeing the same results."

"Yes, that's what I'm seeing in my patients," said Marie.

"When we used the brain of a diseased kuru victim in our frog trials, they died kuru-like deaths. We were just young, eager, and yes, naive scientists bent on discovering something new. We never dreamed it would be used for evil."

"What I've noticed, however," said Marie, "is that from onset of symptoms, the progression of this new insomnia flu is much more rapid than what I have read about FFI."

"Senator Bonner died within six months of her first symptoms," said Jilian, "but she was tougher than most. Even someone as healthy and headstrong as she was . . . six months . . . just so quick."

"Luca can speak to that better than I," started Jacob, "but from what he told me—see if this makes sense, Luca?" Luca nodded. "Some people are homozygotes, and some are heterozygotes. When considering prion diseases, and right now, we're about ninety-nine percent sure that's what we're dealing with - if you're a heterozygote, you have either a smaller chance of getting infected or if you do contract the disease, your progression will be slower."

"You're a good student, Jacob. I think we're seeing something a bit different, however, because very few victims—from reports on medical sites and speaking with Dr. Jimmerson, appear to live longer than six months. There are considerably more heterozygotes in our population, so on the surface, it would appear heterozygosity is your ticket to immunity."

Kira raised her hand.

"I know what you're going to ask," said Jacob. "As you may or may not know, we all have two copies of each gene—one from our father and one from mom. We also have a prion gene. Yep, we all have one. It's called Prion Protein or PRNP."

"I assume this genetics lesson is important for us to know?" asked Jilian.

"Yes, it is," said Luca. "I have tried to bring this down to a level most of you would understand, but to quote Sun Tzu, 'If you know the enemy and know yourself, you need not fear the result of a hundred battles.' To finish what Jacob started, homozygotes have the same amino acid on each of the two prion genes. It's called valine. Heterozygotes have methionine on one and valine on the other. It's this difference which prevents them from getting the insomnia flu, and that's why every fifty-five-year-old you know isn't getting sick."

During Luca's explanation, Jacob received a text from Tom:

We're shutting down for the night.
Printing and circ have the con. Over.

Thanks, Tom. Get something on those eyes.
See you tomorrow.

Printing of the *Arizona Times Herald* was done at their facility downtown on Central Avenue, after which it was trucked to Circulation two blocks over. Jacob had hoped they could consolidate operations into one facility, but COVID caused him to hit the delay button and now he hoped to do so in 2023.

"Enough about genetics. Let's talk about the immediate future. First, as you know, Luca believes he has a way to stop the insomnia flu from progressing in the victims, but it hasn't been trialed yet. We have no time to go through FDA approval—too many lives would be lost by the time it moved through the system. Here's the catch." He glanced at Luca, who nodded in his direction. "Luca will release the solution when he is confident the people who are responsible for the InF will be punished appropriately. I must say I share this wish. Having said that, this is how we—What's that smell?"

62

"Smells like smoke," someone said as they all stood and headed for the door. Jilian was closest and when she opened the door, she could see smoke at the other end of the expansive newsroom. The lights were out, giving the emerging gray fog a chilling personality.

"No elevators!" yelled Jacob, as he saw a few sprinting toward them. He knew in the presence of fire the elevator would descend to the bottom floor automatically and open the doors. This had been in place for many years to protect anyone who might be trapped. *But why aren't the alarms going off?* he thought. *Why are the sprinklers not activated?* "The stairs!"

Using the scant illumination from streetlights outside the eleventh story window, he hurried toward the door on the west side of the office, worried about Luca and his two hundred and sixty pounds of bulk making it down eleven floors. When he reached the door and turned the heated knob, it just spun. When he yanked, the knob pulled out of the door, causing Jacob to lose his balance and fall into Luca behind him. As they peered through the hole, they could see flames beginning to rise from the stairwell.

"Everyone back! The fire is coming up this way. Let's try the elevators now!"

Kyle was already there, and when he got close, he could feel the heat coming through the seams. "Not going to work. Must be fire in the shaft."

"I called 911," Kira said. "They knew about the fire. Said it would be three minutes."

"Are there exterior stairs?" asked Luca.

"We used to have 'em," Kira responded, "but after two break-ins, we got rid of 'em."

Smoke filled the room, and the temperature was now at a dangerous level. They instinctively fell to the floor and searched for air that was easier to breathe. Each pushed aside fatalistic thoughts of calling or texting loved ones. They heard no sirens in the distance.

Jacob saw a text come through on his cell from an unknown number.

> If you're still alive, I want you to know it's nothing
> personal, but when you play with fire . . .

His breathing was labored. Seeing an electric fan at a desk nearby, he tried using it to improve the oxygen in the area by blowing smoke away but found it only recirculated the stagnant air. Six feet over, he saw Luca lying still. *Hang on, Luca. Hang on!* He heard Kira, stumbling and coughing, then could make out her walking toward him. She held a neck scarf over her nose, but he saw no other movement.

A loud explosive sound above his head made him instinctively duck even lower. Sheetrock, ceiling tile, HVAC ductwork and foam insulation rained down, covering him and likely others with dust and insulation fibers. A sudden *whoosh* of smoke was sucked up through the new hole, giving him a short reprieve from what had become a shroud of grayness.

Jacob peered up through cleaner air to see a figure outlined against a moonlit sky. A ladder appeared next to him as he heard shouts from the silhouette.

"Climb up! Hurry!"

63

He moved to a kneeling position and searched for life, then found a prostrate Kira through the haze. He crawled to her, wrapped his hands under her shoulders and dragged her to the ladder. As he approached it, he saw Kyle doing the same with Marie. The air around the ladder was considerably less pungent as the nighttime air above sucked the oxygen-deprived air up and out into the darkened sky. Kira's eyes opened and her new awareness gave her enough strength with Jacob's support to climb the ladder to safety on the roof. Kyle and Marie executed a similar exercise.

As soon as they were out of harm's way, Jacob and Kyle searched for Luca and Jilian. Jacob knew Luca would be difficult to drag if he found him, but no sooner did he get concerned than Luca crawled into view, wheezing, but moving.

"Can't leave me here, guys," he said weakly.

They helped him to the ladder, then supported it while he climbed and rolled onto the roof. Once he knew Luca was safe, he fell prostrate again and began the search for Jilian. Kyle went the opposite direction, but they saw flames engulfing desks and threatening to engulf the entire floor. The temperature steadily rose.

Shouts from the roof came. "Get out of there! Get up the ladder before it's too late! Hurry!"

They ignored the shouts from Kira and Marie.

"Jilian! Jilian! Jilian!"

The flames crept closer. Six feet away now, Kyle and Jacob were on hands and knees at the ladder.

"Jilian!"

As the flames threatened to overtake the ladder, they hurried up the steps to the roof. Exhausted from the escape, they knew there was little time before the roof was engulfed.

Still recovering as she lay on her back, Kira scrutinized the figure that saved their lives. "Sawyer! How did you—"

"Don't worry about that right now. I have a rope long enough so everyone can get off this thing. Women first!" He quickly escorted Kira over to the edge of the building furthest from the elevator and stairs where a rope was tied around an air-conditioning unit.

"Will this hold me?"

"Of course. I have large knots every two feet in the rope. Just go hand over hand, grabbing each knot as you go down. Keep going until you reach the ground. Helps if you close your eyes. You'll be fine."

She took a deep breath and began her descent. Marie followed six feet behind.

Sawyer sent Luca next. "Think you can handle this, big guy?"

The clean air returned Luca's exuberant personality. "I've climbed the three highest mountains in Italy. This is like a kiddie slide!"

Jacob watched as he began the descension with little hesitancy or trouble. "I can feel the heat through the roof," Jacob said. Flames shot through the breach Sawyer created using a block of

C4 and a detonator. "Still don't hear any sirens. We need to get off this roof quickly!"

"Age before beauty and the beast, doctor." Sawyer smirked.

Kyle backed toward the edge of the roof, knowing if he peered over the edge, he might not be able to make the eleven-story journey. He grabbed the rope, eased himself over, closed his eyes and began the sortie.

"I'll be right behind you, Jacob. Go!"

"Sorry, but the captain is always the last one off the ship. I'm not moving until you head down. Besides, I know you can get down faster. By the way, did I ever tell you about the time I got blown off the top of an oil derrick in the Gulf of Mexico and survived?"

"This is hardly the time—"

"I landed in a film of oil. Thirteen others landed in water from sixty yards up and died, but I landed in an oil spill caused by the high winds at the edge of eye. Hurricanes can't even kill me, Sawyer. Now go!"

Sawyer knew it was hopeless, so he followed Kyle. Jacob saw parts of the roof beginning to cave in and prayed the air conditioning unit would not collapse before they were all safely on terra firma. As he glanced over the edge, he could see Sawyer had already made it to the tenth floor, and he could see Kira was already on the ground. He grabbed the rope and began his escape.

As he neared the ninth floor, he saw the far corner of the roof cave in, then flames burst through the windows to his right. Glass rained down on spectators who congregated below. When he neared the eighth, he looked down to see Kira and Marie running across the street, evading gawkers who had little regard for avoiding harm's way. His hands already raw from the strands of the burlap rope knots, he wondered how the ladies had handled this.

He was now at the seventh floor and saw Kira and Marie frantically waving their arms as if the movement would speed up the passage of time. More windows exploded outwardly, as if someone inside was using a blow torch to shatter the glass that continued to fall indiscriminately. The herd below had thinned considerably since the first shower.

By the time he reached the sixth floor, he was close enough to Sawyer to hear him urging Kyle to hurry. He could see Luca on the sidewalk below, scanning the side of the building to check on their progress before he scampered across the street.

When he passed the fifth floor, he heard a loud noise from above, followed by a hard jerk of the rope that pulled him ten feet higher. If he had not been gripping the knot at the time, he could have easily lost his connection to the rope and fallen fifty feet onto bare concrete. *Damn. AC unit must have fallen through the roof.* His shoulders felt like they had taken the brunt of the force and he worried if his repaired rotator cuff would survive the shock. He looked down. "Everyone okay?"

Then he saw Kira and Marie running back across the street toward the building. He picked up his speed, though his shoulders, arms and hands objected. He fell from one knot to the next and knew any minute, the rope wrapped around the air conditioning unit could burn through and release him onto the unforgiving ground below.

At about the fourth floor, he felt the rope give a little and quickly debated whether to crawl into a flameless window and escape another way, but he never stopped his accelerated scramble down the vertical brick wall.

When he reached the third floor, he could finally hear sirens. At the second floor, he could see Luca and the ladies helping Kyle across the street, but a few more knots down, the lifeline finally broke loose and dropped Jacob the final ten feet, just as Sawyer jumped clear. He landed and rolled to avoid some of the shock to his joints.

"Sorry I didn't catch you," said Sawyer, grinning as he helped Jacob up. "It appears our good Dr. Hunter hurt something with that surprise jolt. They crossed the street as two fire trucks drove into view. The others had found an area on the other side of Mont-pelier bank, away from the ogling masses.

"Kyle tore his ACL," said Marie. "We need to get him to a hospital."

"That's risky," said Jacob. "We don't know who, if anyone, was responsible for this. If someone was, they could be watching us. Let's get out of here first. I don't want to get detained by the police and we need to talk to Sawyer." He glanced at the man who had saved them . . . the man who had information he needed.

64

"I told you not to call me until I was out of the city."

"I need assurances." Antioch had heard from the others but needed to hear it from Salamander.

"Watch the news."

"That won't help me. Before you get the second installment, I need details. Details that show you didn't leave any evidence."

Salamander pulled into Airport Parking and tried to remain cool. "My associate will call you in ten minutes. If you want details, you will be by your phone."

Nine minutes later, Antioch's phone buzzed. "Antioch."

A female voice replied with the cadence and emotion of a 1964 IBM Selectric typewriter. "On floor number four of the Century Building at precisely 8:15, Mister X, using gloves and a ski mask, disabled the video feed. He used a Bic lighter and gasoline to start the fire. Furniture that was already on the floor was arranged to ensure the fire would reach the ceiling. He rode the elevator to the tenth floor. He placed a metal bar between the elevator doors to prevent them from closing. He exited through the elevator roof. He lit a rag and tossed it to the bottom of the shaft. He doused the edges of the shaft with gasoline. He threw the two empty cans of gasoline to the bottom of the shaft. He climbed back into the elevator. He exited through the door and removed the bar. He went to the stairwell. He emptied the last can of gasoline as he walked down to the first floor. He left the can on the third step. He used his lighter to ignite the stairs. He left the scene."

The line went dead. Antioch smiled.

65

Across the street from where they had shimmied down the side of an eleven-story building, restaurant patrons, cab drivers and inebriated divorcees from Gatsby's Bar continued to rush or stumble by them, knowing they could tell coworkers tomorrow at the Sparklett's cooler they watched the Century Building burn down. A light sprinkle helped cool off the heat-saturated sidewalks, jazz music played to an empty bar down the block and swaying beams from a grand opening searchlight appeared to ignore the fact a building constructed at the turn of the twentieth century struggled to exist.

Jacob motioned Sawyer to help him walk Kyle, who at four inches taller than Jacob's six-foot-four-inch frame had to lean over to put his arm around the shorter Sawyer.

"Where are we going?" asked Kira.

"There's a CVS two blocks up. Let's get some ibuprofen and a wrap or knee brace for Kyle. From there, I know of a Best Western another block down and have an idea for how we can lose someone if they're watching." Jacob glanced back to see long streams of water coming from the fire trucks shooting through burning windows and onto the roof. He cued up *Stand By You* by Rachel Platten for a gait song, grabbed Kyle around the waist, and headed south to the beat. None of the oncoming rabble cared or even noticed six people walk away from the excitement, assisting an elderly guy with a bum knee while one guy's mind was on a girl named Rachel.

After Kyle downed three ibuprofens, Marie wrapped his knee tightly with an ACE bandage and grinned as he instructed her in the figure-eight technique. They navigated to the Best Western, where Jacob requested an Uber Black SUV pick them up on the corner of Sixth and Magnolia, banking that the bad guys did not have access to Uber data. They exited the hotel onto fifth avenue through the door on the other side, walked another block south and entered Dexter's Bar. Jacob found Dexter, who had advertised in the *Arizona Times Herald* for twenty years and asked if they could leave through the employee's entrance.

Jacob had them wait until the SUV pulled up, then told them to pile in as fast as they could.

The red-cheeked and amiable driver held a black and white shih tzu in his lap. "You Mr. Potter?"

"That's me."

After all were in and the doors closed, the driver said, "Headed to the DoubleTree Suites on Fourth, right?"

"That's right."

"That's pretty close to the Century Building. Did you hear it was burning? It may fall over on that hotel. You sure about that?"

"Very. Thanks, Gustavo."

"I'm here to serve!" he said with a grin, stroking the small dog's head, as he turned onto Wiggans Avenue.

Jacob concluded anyone pursuing them would not search close to the Century Building, assuming they would want to get as far from the source of the attempted murder as they could. As they drove the few short blocks, Jacob reflected it was not only attempted murder, but if Jilian had not made it out alive, as he feared, they had killed already. He would not allow them to add to the number.

After Gustavo deposited them at the DoubleTree, they found an unoccupied sitting area. They saw only the receptionist.

"Did you ever see Jilian?" asked Kira, hoping against hope to hear something good. Jacob and Kyle shook their heads and returned Kira's glance through sorrowful eyes.

"We didn't hear her either," said Jacob. "I'm not sure what happened . . . why she got separated. Did anyone see her go in another direction?"

They all appeared equally confused. "It was difficult to see anything in there, and I had my eyes closed to keep the smoke from burning," said Marie. "I hope she found another way out." She checked her phone. "Nothing from her yet."

"Kyle, you okay for now?" asked Jacob. "We need Sawyer to answer some questions for us."

Kyle nodded. "I'm good."

Jacob glanced toward the front desk and saw a pear-shaped middle-aged woman with makeup two shades shy of a clown face striding toward them. He worried she would ask them to move on.

"Did you guys know about the Century Building burning? It's why you don't see anyone here. They all took off to see the fire. Ain't it amazing how that attracts people like a dead cow attracts buzzards?"

"Ma'am, we're from out of town," said Marie. "We're having a committee meeting. Is it okay if we sit here for a spell? Mr. Stone here hurt his knee and needed a break." Kyle waved at her.

"Why sure, honey. Just let me know if you want something from the bar. Tiffini done run out with all the vultures . . . I mean customers, to see the light show, but I tended bar for ten years."

"Why thank you, Collette," said Marie. "Can we just have some water for now?"

"Sure thing, sweetie. Ain't got nothing better to do right now." She waddled off to the bar.

"Sawyer." Jacob turned toward him, as did the others. A cheap chandelier above them flickered annoyingly. "First, we can't thank you enough for saving our lives. I won't downplay that now or ever. I know the ladies have already hugged you, but I wanted to say that for the men here." Sawyer nodded, knowing what was coming next.

"I think one question will satisfy most of our curiosity. How did you come to be on the roof and have a rope ready to save our butts? You have the floor."

Sawyer leaned forward, elbows on his knees. Moisture seeped from his cobalt eyes. "They have my boys."

66

The group gave him a puzzled look. "Who is 'they'?" asked Kira.

Sawyer shook his head. "I don't know, exactly. I got a text from someone a week ago that said my boys were in danger, and the only way to save them was to do a job for them. I was to drop off my sons at my sister's house . . . I didn't want to involve her, but I really had no choice."

"Do you know why they used you?" asked Jacob.

Sawyer hung his head and answered from a posture of shame. "They used me before. Paid me a hundred thousand to make sure you knew about Ted's phone being in his locker—then I had to take Kira to the address of a lady who supposedly had one of the plants."

"You were acting strange that day," Kira said with a hint of disdain.

"I thought I covered well, but you can usually see through my shit. Anyway, when I got to the door, the lady who opened it gave me an envelope. When she knew my name, I wasn't surprised at that point. Felt like I was being watched." Sawyer avoided Kira's stare.

Collette walked up with a tray of waters for the group. "Here you are, but from what I can see, what you really need are some stiff drinks, and I know you ain't drivin' tonight." She laid the tray of waters on the glass table between them.

"Thank you, Collette," said Kira. "This will be fine for now."

"I move we help fund the adult beverage industry at the conclusion of the committee meeting," said Luca.

"Second!" Marie responded, drawing an eye from Jacob.

"All in favor?"

All but Jacob raised their hands. "Motion carries."

Collette rolled her eyes and found her way back to the reception desk.

"What was in the envelope?" asked Kira.

"I didn't open it until you dropped me off. It had some long-range telephoto images of my boys at recess. That's all that was in there. Then I got the text later that day."

"What was the job?" asked Jacob.

"My instructions were to wait for a bag to be delivered to my front door. Then I was to take the bag to a house on Carpenter in Chandler but was to park on Dempsey. There was a remote in the bag I was to use to open the garage door, then replace the bulb in the ceiling with one from the bag."

"Did they tell you what this was all about? Whose house it was?" asked Jacob.

"No, and I didn't ask. Didn't think they would tell me anyway, and I didn't want to upset 'em."

"His story checks out," said Kira.

Sawyer gave her a puzzled expression. "How did—"

"I followed you."

"You what?"

"I didn't mean to. When you called in sick, I got worried about you and was going to your house to see if I could get you anything, and when I saw you driving away . . . when you reported a hundred and four degree-temperature, my curiosity demanded I follow you. Can't control that."

"Then you saw me go to the airport?"

"Yes. You were flying to Milan, Italy."

"Those were my instructions. The reservation information was in the bag."

"That was a quick trip," said Marie.

"I never went. They wanted me to leave the country, but I couldn't leave with my boys in danger. No way. After I was seated on the plane, I pretended to go to the bathroom in first class while people were still getting on. When I came out of the bathroom, I turned right and headed back up the jet bridge and when an agent asked what I was doing, I said I had to buy some Tums, but would be right back and to be sure and save my seat. 'Name is Noah Settle,' I told them. I saw that name on the guy's ticket in front of me."

"Did you think they were watching you?" asked Jacob.

"I don't know, but wasn't taking any chances, and if they were on to me after that, they would've already . . . well, I don't know what they would've done. I sat in Chile's for about an hour, then took a cab to my sister's house."

"The one in Scottsdale?"

"Yes—Bailey's house, because that's where they told me to take Derrall and Weldon. They said they had someone there who'd be watching 'em . . . making sure I did my job."

"The house you were sent to change the light bulb in blew up," said Kira, "and the young woman who lived there was an atmospheric chemist. She was working with a Harvard microbiologist on what they called a real-time vaccination—one that could stop and even reverse the effects of an infected insomnia flu victim."

"Oh God . . . did . . . did . . . she survive?" Drops of perspiration dripped from his temples and his face lost even more color in the light of the overhead chandelier.

"She's in a medically induced coma right now. She developed a lot of swelling on the brain from what they told me, and this would help. I'm sure Marie or Kyle could explain it better."

"That must mean her head was injured," Kyle said. "In any injury, there's usually swelling, and this decreases the blood flow to the area, which of course reduces oxygen as well, so they induce a coma to allow the brain to rest. It decreases the brain's electrical activity and metabolic rate, so over time, this allows the swelling to subside."

"They said something about a drain," said Kira.

"That helps reduce the swelling also," offered Marie. "It's pretty common. I hope she recovers."

"They told me they hope it wouldn't cause long-term damage," said Kira, "but either way, she's lost a leg and an eye."

"Wait," said Luca. "What is her name?"

"Dr. Ludmila Porphyr."

67

"Oh no. I was afraid of that. There aren't that many atmospheric chemists in the world. She was a grad student at Padua when Enzo and I were doing our experiments with prion aerosols."

Sawyer hung his head. He couldn't look at Kira or anyone else.

After a moment, Marie broke the uncomfortable silence. "They had your boys, Sawyer. You had no choice."

"Yes, I did . . . I could've called the police, even though they warned me not to."

"I'm glad you didn't," exhorted Jacob. "That would've been a bad move."

Marie checked her phone again for anything from Jilian, but nothing had come in except for a few messages from her team. Her office manager told her Elizabeth was going to make it. The gun shot from one of the two men missed vital organs.

Kyle propped his wrapped leg onto an empty chair and hoped the new angle would soften the discomfort he was feeling after the ibuprofen wore off. "Back to the roof, Sawyer. How—?"

"Okay," Sawyer eagerly said, relieved to move the conversation in a different direction. "After I left the airport, like I said, I went to my sister's house."

"Left your car at the airport?" asked Kyle.

"Yes, in case they were making sure I didn't take a flight back and take it. I didn't know what to expect at my sister's house after they had said someone was watching my boys, so I had the cab drop me off a block away and went down the alley to the back of the house."

"Was it still daylight?" asked Kira.

"It was dusk by the time I got there. I stayed in the alley behind some trash cans. Watched for about twenty minutes but never saw any movement. When it got dark, I was able to see through some windows, and Jacob, you're not going to believe who I saw."

"Ted."

"How did you know?"

"I was told Ted had only one sister who had died. But then his sister picked him up from the office. Ran a check on Ted's history using his social. We didn't go back far enough when we hired him, but he was a securities broker and a B actor in some movies you never heard of. None of that pointed to a mailroom guy."

"But how did you know he would be at my sister's house?"

"The building's security cameras. We reviewed the recordings from the day she picked him up—think it was last Thursday—we got her license plate. Traced to an address in Peoria. I hired Capri—"

"Where'd you uncover *him*?" asked Kira.

"When we did that human-interest story on him a few years ago, I saved his cell number. You never know, right?" He grinned, and Kira nodded. "You know how good he is, so I paid him to flush her out. He told her she could stay out of trouble if she told him where she took Ted. He was very . . . convincing. I just got this information yesterday, so when you mentioned your sister lived in Scottsdale, the pieces fell together."

"When I saw Ted talking on the phone," Sawyer continued, "I had an idea. My sister inherited that house from my parents back in ninety-two. We grew up there and used to crawl under the house—it was a pier and beam type, so there was a small door in the back of the house we could crawl through and listen through the floor to our parents talking. We used to keep an old beer glass down there to help us listen and it was still there. Kira knows about this too—"

"I thought you might mention that," Kira said.

"Yeah, it's an app called *Amplitude* that helps to hear conversations more clearly. We didn't have it back then, but Kira and I have used it to listen in . . . never mind. Not important. Anyway, there was a lot of shouting and screaming back then, but we could hear them even when they weren't fighting."

Kira's mind wandered to her own childhood. Her dad's job as a detective took him away much of the time, but when he was home, she never remembered her parents fighting. She and her sister, Karla, were challenging at times, but Kira's admiration for her father kept her in line.

"So, what did you hear Ted saying?"

"That's how I found out about their plans to burn the Century Building. I could only hear Ted's part of the conversation, but I caught enough to hear they knew about your meeting, and the plan was for no one to survive. Ted was to help a guy named Salamander, who had already placed desks, chairs, and boxes in a pile in the middle of the fourth floor, then soaked them with gasoline."

"That floor's been vacant since COVID," said Jacob.

"Must be why they chose it," said Sawyer. "Ted was to ride up to the ninth floor at seven and wait for a message."

"You picked up quite a bit from hearing one side of that conversation," Kyle said.

"It was obvious to me the person on the other end of the line was having Ted repeat back everything he said to make sure he understood. What I understood quickly is Ted never had the insomnia flu."

"You saw no sign of your boys? Or your sister?" asked Kyle.

"That was the last thing they discussed," Sawyer said as his eyes moistened. He took a few seconds to compose himself. "He had a gun. . . he had a gun."

68

"Did he do something with it?" Luca asked, showing some frustration with the slow unraveling of the story mixed with the tragic end of a normal life for Dr. Ludmila Porphyr.

"It was *his* gun!" Sawyer said forcefully.

"I'm sure it was," said Kyle. "What aren't you telling us?"

Sawyer's head dropped. The others waited anxiously. When he finally lifted his head, he appeared more resolute. "Ted said to whoever was on the phone 'They've been . . . taken care of.'"

"Are you sure he was talking about your boys?" asked Marie.

"I was pretty sure, since I didn't see any sign of them, but wanted to make sure. There was another crawl space and door from under the house that opened into the garage. I didn't know what I would do with it, but I found a crowbar in the dark. I pressed the garage door opener and stood with my back to the wall by the door that led into the kitchen. In a few seconds, I saw the door open, and an arm come through it, holding that gun. He started to look toward me when I came down with the crowbar . . . I think I broke his arm, and the gun flew a few feet away. It's like he didn't even care about his arm because he came at me and used his left arm to shove me back into some golf clubs. I was lying on the floor and tried to pick up an iron to defend myself, but he was already on me."

"Ted must go at least three-fifty," said Jacob.

"I felt it. I got an elbow free and rammed it into the broken arm, then used my knee to get him in the groin. When he rolled over in pain, I crawled over to the gun and pointed it at him. I'd never shot a gun before, and he could probably tell I didn't know what I was doing. I told him to lay there and not get up or I would shoot. I told him to tell me where my boys were. He didn't say anything at first—just stared at me and got up. I asked him again where my boys were, but he started walking toward me. I told him I would shoot, but that didn't stop him. Before he grabbed the gun, I pulled the trigger. There was blood everywhere." Sawyer shook his head. "Now I may never find out where my boys are . . . or even if they're alive."

Marie thought of something. "Sawyer!" When he turned to her, she pulled a piece of paper from her pocket and unfolded it. She turned it toward him. "Did you happen to see a design like this on Ted?" During their meeting in the Century Building, she doodled out a picture of the graphic she had seen on the motorcyclist's wrist during her chilling bike ride the week before. It resembled the outline of a genie in baggy clothes laying on her side.

"Yes!" he said, "but what's this about?"

"I had a warning from a few . . . let's say undesirables when I biked from Kyle's place last week. They scared the-you-know-what out of me and said they would always know where I was. Not sure I believe them, but I took it as a sign I'm—or we—could be on the right track."

"Why didn't you tell me?" asked Kyle, reproachfully.

"They told me not to. I couldn't take a chance on putting you in danger. That's why I left the next day. But I knew I had seen that mark somewhere else, and it hit me yesterday. The guard outside Jilian's room had the same mark."

Kira moved next to Sawyer during his recounting and placed her arm around him. "We'll find your boys, Sawyer. I know they're alive . . . and so is your sister." He had his face in his hands and Kira could feel him shaking.

"Sawyer," Jacob said hesitantly. "I know this might not be the best time, but what did you do with the body? Are you sure he was dead?"

Sawyer's head hung. "I didn't even think to check. There was so much blood . . . and he wasn't moving. Maybe I was in shock. I don't know. I was aware enough to realize my sister's car wasn't in the garage, but I had blood all over me and all I could think of was to get clean. To get the memory off me. I found some car keys in his pocket. He had a Miata out front, so I drove it to my house to take a shower and clear my head."

"So is the body still in the garage?" asked Luca.

Sawyer nodded. "I haven't been back. I guess so."

"You didn't bring his phone, did you?" asked Jacob.

"I did at first. Thought I would have some time to think about the best thing to do on the drive to my house, and about halfway home, I decided to get rid of it. I found a drain hole in the side of the street and chunked it in after I made sure no one was watching."

"Were there any homes or businesses nearby that could have filmed it on their cameras?" asked Kyle.

"I thought about that and made sure. It was on Eleventh, I think. Yes, Eleventh."

"Good move, Sawyer. If they trace it, they'll have fun down in the sewer, combing through the sludge."

"Ted's car shouldn't be at your house," Marie warned.

"I decided that too, after I was clean and had some time to think. I cleaned the steering wheel and door handles and put on gloves. I knew I didn't want to get my car at the airport, so last night, I called one of my golf buddies. Owns a pickup he never drives, and he let me borrow it. I told him to meet me at the spot we used to fish at on the Gila River. I left the Miata there and took him back to his house in Arondale. When I came up this afternoon, I left it about two blocks from our office . . . on McDowell."

69

Collette wandered back over, anticipating the committee meeting was over and hoping she could extract some drink orders from the group. By this point, they were ready to order something to both get their minds off recent tragedies and to celebrate their escape from attempted murder. She took their orders and hurried over to the bar. A few people began to filter back in. Conversations universally revolved around the fire and two men were making nonmonetary bets on whether the building would be leveled or resurrected once the fire was extinguished.

"I assume you didn't go to the police with any of this?" asked Kyle.

"I considered it, but I thought if the information got into the wrong hands, they would eliminate me . . . then I wouldn't have been any help to my boys or to you guys. If I made an anonymous call, they wouldn't believe me, and even if they did—"

"They might have at least checked it—"

"Besides, Kira" Sawyer interrupted, "I thought if I could get you out of there without them knowing, we would have an advantage. Selfishly, I wanted your help finding my boys . . . and sister."

"But the building?" Jacob asked.

"I called the management company from Ted's phone before I tossed it into the sewer. I pretended like I was an agent wanting to sell them property insurance. Said 'you never know when a fire or flood could destroy the building'. They told me they already had coverage for Acts of God and vandalism."

"That was some clear thinking, Sawyer. I know we have contents insurance for our office and all information is stored on the cloud, so all in all, I think you made the right decisions."

"Get to the rope," implored Kira.

"Ah yes. Remember the stunt we covered a few years ago by the stunt double for Angelina Jolie?"

"Eloise Fordham."

"That's her."

"I thought I remembered that rope from somewhere."

"Yep," said Sawyer. "She used it to climb two hundred feet up to a helicopter, getting in just as it flew over Chase Tower. Anyway, I remembered asking her where she stored a rope that long between stunts and she told me about her storage facility outside of Scottsdale. I told her I needed to borrow it for a Kiwanis Club tug-of-war. Told her we would give her some cred."

"How did you get it to the roof?" asked Kyle.

"You know those big mail carts we have at the—"

"You mean *had*," said Jacob.

"Yeah, I doubt they survived. I loaded one up with the rope and took it up the elevator at a little after noon today. That only got it to the eleventh floor, so the hard part was taking it up the set of stairs to the roof. No one ever uses the stairs, so I had plenty of time to pull it up."

"And the explosive?" asked Luca. "That had to be powerful to blow through the roof and then the ceiling."

"C4."

"Where did you get C4?" asked Kyle. "I thought only the armed forces could get that."

"The armed forces and those involved in underwater seismic charges. I've been dating a girl who's working on a project in the Caribbean to study the hydroacoustic, seismic and acoustic effects of underwater explosions on the reef's ecosystem. I know that's a mouthful, but she made me memorize that, so I didn't mess it up when I talked to people and make them think she was blowing up fish."

"And she was using C4 to simulate other explosions?" asked Kira.

"Yes. Reagan's spending time in Scottsdale after her brother died . . . just to take some time off, but she helped me acquire some for the job."

"What did you tell her you were going to use it for?" asked Jacob.

"Told her I was going to blow a hole in the Century Building. She just rolled her eyes and didn't ask again."

70

Collette placed the drinks for everyone on the glass table and received the appropriate appreciation. After she walked away, Jacob raised his glass of the house cabernet and said, "To Jilian, who we pray found a way to freedom, and to Sawyer, who granted us ours." They clinked their glasses in somber unity.

A committee decision was made to make the DoubleTree their temporary domicile for the night. They felt fortunate there were available rooms with Bruno Mars playing at Comerica Theatre nearby. Kyle had a debit card he used to pay for the six rooms. They checked in as the extended Stone family: Peter, Rock, Larry, Joshua, Alice, and Lynette. They agreed to meet at 7:30 in the morning in room 418. "I'm up at five-thirty every morning, so I'll have bagels and coffee ready for everyone," said Jacob. What he failed to mention was he wanted to walk over to his former place of business before the sunrise awoke Phoenix. It would give him a chance to survey the landscape, and maybe, just maybe discover an answer to Jilian's disappearance. This would be easy, as he had not slept well the past few days. He decided not to let the others know about the plant his wife brought into their marriage that smelled so sweet.

Jacob had one last message for the group. "We don't know if those who would do us harm are aware of our escape or not, but the best course of action is for us to assume they are unaware. I say that to say this. No one should communicate with anyone outside our group this evening. Don't reply to any texts and don't answer your phones. I know you have family who're worried. I do too, but this group already killed Danny King and Darcy Sandam . . . and maybe Jilian. They've ruined the life of a doctor who was getting close to an answer for InF, burnt down a building in an attempt to exterminate all of us here, and if they're responsible for the four hundred and thirty-eight thousand InF deaths so far, they won't allow anyone to get in their way. But we can't just run. More lives are at stake. With Luca's help, we have a plan we'll discuss in the morning in detail. You all stink and need baths soon, so I'll see you in the morning."

As the others headed for the elevator, Jacob grabbed Sawyer's arm and pulled him aside.

"Listen, I wanted to thank you again for the bravery you showed today. I know you want to find your boys and sister, and we will help you, but the plan tomorrow needs to happen first. Do you understand?" Sawyer nodded reluctantly. "I assume you've tried to contact your sister?"

He nodded again. "I'm scared."

"I know," said Jacob. "I know."

"Hey, did you really fall off an oil derrick?"

Jacob grinned. "I'm afraid of heights. You'd never get me up on one of those."

71

Zermatt, Switzerland

"Yes, I read online about the Century Building. That tells me nothing."

"Relax, Antioch. I held up the fire department for seven minutes, just as you said. You were right, by the way. When I told Sargent Salters to stay the order because it was an arson fraud case, he was happy to see the criminals lose everything."

"Any survivors? And where are you right now, Poseidon?"

"Too early to tell about survivors, but I would say there's little chance. Salamander disabled the elevator and stairs. We received a 911 call from inside the building, but that was rerouted. Started the fire in the middle of the fourth floor after disarming the alarms, so no flames were seen until the interior of the building was toast. He knows what he's doing."

"Did he hang around to make sure?"

"Antioch. He's a professional. He's *the* professional. Says he's not a pyromaniac who gets gratification in witnessing the aftermath. By the time the fire was out tonight, he was on a plane to Lisbon."

"You didn't tell me where you are," Antioch said impatiently.

"New Orleans. At the IACP International Meeting. I needed to be out of Phoenix."

"And Falcon?"

"Visiting his daughter in Springfield, Missouri."

"I don't like this. Doesn't feel right."

"It's fine, Antioch. I fly back in the morning. I'll give you a status update then. You're nine hours ahead of us there. I'll keep that in mind. Oh, one more thing. You lost any hair lately?"

"What the hell is that supposed to mean?"

"Nothing. Just curious."

72

Phoenix, Arizona

The next morning, Jacob walked past the night receptionist, whose eyes were glued to the latest issue of *People* magazine and walked into the still and dimly lit sidewalks lining the street. Just ahead, smoldering remains sent afterthoughts of an extinguished fire into the pre-dawn sky. Soon, the dark would fade, and the cool whispers of an easterly breeze would give way to the unrelenting and unrepentant sun. He could see forklifts, a crane, and a Sky Track telehandler among the remains. One forklift was at work along with search lights scanning for evidence of life. He watched a gray-bearded stocky man in soot-covered overalls sit on a bench and remove his hard hat to wipe the perspiration from his hairless scalp.

"Been a long night?" Jacob asked as he sat beside him.

The question startled the older man, but he recovered quickly. Turning his head toward Jacob, he eyed him for a second, then said, "Don't think you're supposed to be here. That yellow—"

"My brother was in that building."

"I'm sorry, Mr. . . ."

"Collins. Gary Collins." Jacob used the name of his eighth grade history teacher.

"They didn't give us no names, Mr. Gary Collins. Been pullin' collapsed brick and stone out of that pile." He pointed his thumb over his left shoulder at what remained of Jacob's former place of business. "Been careful not to cause any cave-ins. Sure your brother didn't get out?"

Jacob shook his head and forced a tear to escape from his right eye, enabled by lingering smoke. "I've been calling and texting him. He would have communicated with me by now."

"Sorry, Mr. Gary Collins. We were told there could be six bodies. That's how many are unaccounted for. Would your brother be one of 'em?"

"I don't know about any six, Mr. . . ."

"Jessup. I'm Fennimore Jessup, but my friends call me Fenny."

"You're my new friend, Mr. Jessup. Fenny it is. Not sure about the six. Just my brother . . . well, actually, my half-brother. Haven't seen Jacob in twelve years. I was going to surprise him with a visit. Guess I was one day late."

"Fenny! Break's over!" A faceless voice boomed over a pile of burnt sheetrock.

"Sorry, Mr. Gary Collins. Back to Leroy. That's my machine." He rose stiffly and held his back until he was more or less erect. As he trudged back to his telehandler, Jacob called to him.

"Fenny! Have you found any bodies yet?"

He turned forty-five degrees and shook his head. Jacob could read the regret in his non-verbal message.

"Not yet. Building pancaked, so it might be a few days before we get everything moved enough. Sorry again about your brother, Mr. Gary Collins."

After he purchased pigs-in-a-blankets and four dozen holes

from Mimi's Donuts, he found a 7-Eleven and bought six black coffees. Phoenix was now yawning as it threatened to put its feet on the floor and rub the sleepy out of its eyes. The indifferent millennial was on her phone as he walked back by the reception desk at the DoubleTree, laden with the group's nourishment.

She glanced up and said, "We've got free coffee here in the breakfast bar."

"Thanks," said Jacob as he headed for the elevator. "I'll keep that in mind."

"Check-out's at eleven!" he heard her warn as the doors closed and took him to the fourth floor.

73

The group began to arrive at seven-twenty. Marie and Kira walked in together.

How do females always do that? Jacob wondered.

Kyle was next, then Sawyer.

Luca was five minutes late. "Jet lag," he said.

Jacob started. "I don't think I need to remind you the information shared this morning is not to be repeated to anyone. And, to repeat what I said last night, no communication with family and friends. We are all dead. Presumed dead, anyway. At least for forty-eight hours."

"What's the forty-eight hours about?" asked Kyle.

"That's how long it will take them to clear the debris and declare anyone is missing. When they don't recover any bodies—and God I hope they don't recover Jilian's, the manhunt will begin, so that's our window."

"No messages from Jilian," said Marie, whose phone was glued to her hand, "so maybe they'll find one body."

"I don't want to sound uncaring," Jacob responded. "We all hope she's safe somewhere, but we can't dwell on a situation over which we have no control. No time for that. Luca, I'm turning to you now to lay out the plan. I know Marie and Kyle may be able to follow your dive into microbiology, but for the rest of us, especially me, we need you to cliff-note it into a third-grade level."

Luca nodded. "Will do, boss. As you know, there is a group of three men, calling themselves the Klavian Triumvirate, who many years ago left the Zero Population Group and used us—"

"Wait," Kira interrupted. "Who is *us?*"

"I'm referring to Enzo, Artimus, and me. We were all graduate students studying in Italy at the time. They—I mean the Trium-verate—used our work with airborne prion transmissions to create a company we now know as Brand New Horizons, or BNH." He nodded at Kyle. "Dr. Hunter there is responsible for uncovering that detail."

"I'm not sure how it will help us," Kyle said.

"I'm afraid he's right," offered Sawyer. "I found no trace of them after hours of research. It's like they never existed."

"It's probably who has your sons . . . and who's been threat-ening you," Jacob said. He immediately regretted his disclosure.

"I know I'll find them. They're all right." A strained smile crossed Sawyer's face.

Luca continued. "BNH, or whatever they call themselves these days, would ultimately mail prion-infected plants to every-one on their thirty-third birthday. They did this for about seven years, from what we've been able to determine through inter-views."

"From what I've come across in my research," said Marie, "respiratory transmission was not a pathway for the prion causing family familial insomnia."

"They buried our research," Luca lamented. "We didn't know why back then. In fact, from what I recall now, I don't think we even knew they sat on it, but we didn't trust them, so we provided some insurance."

Sunlight propelled through the blinds in the hotel room, and when Jacob saw Luca shielding his eyes, he jumped up to close them. Although they each cleaned up from their descension from the rooftop the day before, they wore the same smoke-saturated clothes in various states of disrepair. Marie's white slacks were closer to gray, and with a button missing from her maroon shirt, she stayed busy preventing exposure of her bra. The desk at the Double Tree had failed to locate a safety pin for her.

Kyle's khaki pants had been ripped by Marie to help get his knee wrapped; Jacob nursed a cut on his chin that opened again; Sawyer found three slivers of glass embedded in his arm and chest, leaving a red target over his heart; Luca had bathed in sweat, giving his pale blue oxford a mottled appearance after drying, and even Kira, who never appeared disheveled, even during a Phoenix monsoon season, had a few tears in her long-sleeved crepe blouse and chic black pants.

After giving a nod to Jacob for blotting out the sun, Luca continued. "As grad students, we had a meager budget, but that didn't stop us from playing around with all kinds of bugs, leeches, fungi, viruses and other parasitic organisms."

"I did that when I was six," Sawyer said.

Kira rolled her eyes at the comment.

"Yeah, I did, too, but we were a bit more educated by that time. We would take these parasites from the Lompoul Desert in Senegal and introduce them to animals who were resident to Italy. We were curious if evolutionary winnowing had created this allopatry, leading—"

"Allopatry? Luca, for God's sake," Kira pleaded.

"It's the word we use for two organisms living in different geographical areas. Anyway, we wanted to see if this evolutionary process had separated the hunter from the hunted. For example, how would a speckled salamander hold up against Scaphiopus couchii?"

"Do I need to get me some popcorn or go grab a degree in animal behavior?" Sawyer asked.

"Sorry. I'm getting to the important part. We mixed and matched for about six months and found reactions that were hard to believe. Death, of course, but some unusual effects occurred—like a Corsican hare that became cannibalistic. We found REM Behavior Disorder in the Italian wolf, tumor growth in the Appenine yellow-bellied toad and suicidal behavior in the Calabrian black squirrel. We had never seen this in the animal kingdom outside of humans, so we knew we were onto something."

"I'm having difficulty connecting any dots here," said Marie, as she fussed with her uncooperative blouse.

"We found one called Bongyloides stercoralis. It's found a few feet under the ground near the Natraria retusa shrub in the Moghra Oasis. It feeds on the root system of the plant but doesn't kill it because the roots regrow within days. It's a symbiotic behavior because the root that regrows is longer and stronger than the one consumed by the parasite."

"Third grade, Luca," Jacob said. "Third grade."

Luca ignored the comment and continued. "We wanted to see what this little bongyloid would do to our animal collection, but when we introduced the critter into the cages of nutria, finches, hares, squirrels, fruit flies, toads and wolves, nothing happened. However, some of these little guys got into the food source, and within twenty hours, our rabbits lost all their hair. Same thing with the nutria. Once we saw this, we brought in marmots, beavers, heck even skunks—same thing. Ever seen a hairless skunk? Possibly the ugliest animal on the planet."

"Did you ever figure out how this was happening?" asked Kyle.

"We were only able to come up with theories, but the best guess is these guys were getting into the blood stream and travelling to the hair bulb of the follicles. We assume they have an affection for this, perhaps feeding on the papilla and killing the follicles."

Marie spoke up before others could. "If we could get those guys to limit their range and direct them to specific areas, count me in for some beta testing." This brought some comic relief to those struggling to stay focused. After a tense eighteen hours, they needed some release.

"Sure these guys aren't Brazilian?" Kira added.

This brought more smiles and admiration for the women who could bring levity to a difficult situation.

It was not clear if Luca appreciated the departure or understood the humor, but he trudged on. "We couldn't stop at the skunk. We slipped some of the parasites into the orangutan's food at the Parco Natura Viva Zoo. We went back the next day, and they were no longer in the open cages. We asked enough questions that we finally were told they had lost their chest and pubic hair. They even brought in psychologists that morning because the animals were distraught."

"All right," said Kira. "This was all fun until you did this to our ancestors."

"No, no. We had our reasons. We were pretty sure either these little guys had eaten their fill or that the circulatory pattern was limited. You probably won't like this, but we went to two other zoos and found the same result. It created a panic in the Veneto region, but I think you'll forgive me when I fill you in on how we plan to use this information."

Luca and Jacob spent the next twenty minutes outlining the plan which needed to happen in the next forty-eight hours.

At 9:36 a.m., they left room number 418 one by one. Jacob called
Tom Bowlsby to arrange a make-shift office in a sparsely leased
three-story brick building on thirty-eighth, which included a
seldom-used workout facility in the basement. They each took
alternate routes to walk there. Sawyer picked up the car he left on
McDowell before camping out on the roof of the Century Building. After consulting with Kyle on a back entrance to the hospital,
Luca took the first step in their action plan by taking a taxi to visit
Dr. Ludmila Porphyr.

74

Tom Bowlsby took everyone's orders for clothes, and after loading up at the Urban Outfitters on Washington Street, dropped them off at the building on thirty-eighth. As instructed, he also brought his laptop from home and a few buckets of chicken from KFC. They spent the next eight hours preparing stories to print and working out details on the plan, with only short breaks to snack and use a bathroom with a defective lock on the door.

Luca returned from talking to Dr. Porphyr in the hospital shortly after 5:00 p.m. and using information she shared, they tweaked the stories and refined the details for the next day. Tom contacted the print shop manager and told him to get the troops in because there would still be an edition going out in the morning. At 9:05 Jacob uploaded the layout and copy for the abridged Monday morning edition of the *Arizona Times Herald.* By 9:25 he had emailed two of the twelve stories they had written to the Associated Press, Reuters, and thirty of the top online news entities. At 9:30, he told everyone to get some sleep wherever they could because Tom would have the van ready by 5:30 a.m. for the trip to Tucson.

"Kira, your sister is on for tomorrow?"

"She's itching to help us. She'll be waiting for us."

75

In a COVID-abandoned building previously leased by the French-owned Friendly Che-Valet, a young woman with matted hair draped over her facial features sat slumped in a wooden rocking chair. Her lips peeled from desiccation as a fan blew warm air from her left, and her tongue lost its ability to moisten. Speech was laborious, but she had little more to say, even if she was capable.

A tall, waifish man entered the concrete room, containing nothing but the rocker and a chair which was currently folded and leaning against the wall. Footprints from previously installed cubicles and desks were evidenced in the dusty floor. Entering through a door to her left, he stood behind her for a moment and nursed a cigar, which was well past its prime. The woman, if she realized his presence, made no indication she did.

He stepped on a rocker rail, causing her body to lurch back, her head flopping reflexively, until he slapped his right hand over her forehead and glared down at her through smoke-colored eyes. She knew those eyes . . . *those eyes* . . . but the dehydration created memory loss.

He allowed the cigar stub to fall, glance off her lips and onto the floor. She did not respond.

"You have been most uncooperative, Ms. Quito. Or should I call you Jilian? I do so hate to be boorish." He increased the pressure with his hand.

She struggled to focus as her airway was compromised, her lungs deprived of oxygen. She would have thrown up after the sudden shift in her bodily position if she had anything to clear out. She made no effort to reply.

He took his foot off the rocker rail and released her head. She inhaled deeply, in anticipation of another unpleasant exercise. If her wrists had not been lashed to the arm rests, she would have been thrown forward onto the cement floor.

"Would you like some water?" he asked as the rocker slowed and he moved around to face her.

Head bowed, she weekly nodded. The man's feral grin would have repelled Jilian if she had seen it. He produced a glass of water and slowly poured it out onto the floor.

"You will tell me what you refused to tell my colleague. I don't know who you have left to protect. Every person in that building is dead."

Jilian looked up to face her antagonist, and in that instant, recognition surfaced. Out of the parched landscape of her oral cavity, she painfully and haltingly said, "I . . . thought . . . you were . . . dead."

This time, she saw the offensive grin. "My poor wife played the part well. It's too bad you got caught in the crossfire. That little explosion was meant for Darcy. You were lucky, but if you continue your silence, you'll wish you'd been crushed in that pile of rubble like my ex-wife. Is that what you call your wife if she's been murdered? No matter."

"How . . . could you . . . do that . . . to your wife?"

He laughed maniacally for what felt to Jilian like minutes. "I don't guess she told you. We were only married for three years, and I told her I was impotent. I needed a cover—"

"For . . . your . . . homosexual behav—"

A sudden punishing slap across her face created enough force to tip the rocking chair without making it topple. Jilian could not rub the throbbing cheek with bound hands, but she was strong enough mentally to hold back any tears. That would signal a lack of resolve. Once she recovered, she sat straight with her chin up as if to say, "do your worst."

"I couldn't stand that bitch. I was only home for a day or two a month, but enough about me. This is about . . . wait, before we leave this, just who knows about my relationship with Albert Leto?"

She shook her head slowly. "No one."

"Now we're getting somewhere." He dragged the folding chair over from the wall and sat in front of her. "A little more information, and you might get a drink of water." He took a large gulp from a glass and wiped his lips as some water dribbled down his chin. "Now, where is the reversal agent kept?"

Once again, she shook her head. "I . . . don't know . . . what you're—"

Another slap. This one from the other side and with a little more force, but again, the chair remained upright. And again, she held back tears which struggled to escape.

"What was your meeting about?" He took another swig from his glass.

"The . . . fire . . . interrupted—"

"Before the fire. Before you tried escaping through the window." He threw what was left in his water glass across her face and she moistened her tongue before the fan had a chance to blow away the drops on her lips. Her mind was jumbled, her memory questionable. She knew she needed to say something believable, so she began.

"We took . . . a vote . . . decided . . . to go . . . to . . . the police . . . with . . . information . . . we learned."

"Which was?" he pressed.

She vainly attempted a swallow, making a show of the effort. This bought her some time to consider her response. "How . . . you did it . . . with the . . . plants."

"Who did what? I hardly believe any of you knew."

"The Klavian . . . Triumvirate," she said resolutely, as she stared into the cold eyes of Kevin Sandam.

"Where is the reversal agent?"

"I told you—" That was all she could get out before Sandam hit her with enough force to knock over the rocking chair. Jilian's arm was pinned under the arm rest and her head caromed off the hard floor. She blacked out, and when she regained consciousness—she was not sure how long it had been—she felt blood soaking the hair beneath her ear and a stinging abrasion on her left cheek. Kevin Sandam was gone.

76

Flagstaff, Arizona

"This better be good news, Falcon." Antioch was not in the mood for anything but.

Falcon squirmed in his chair on the other end of the call. "I'll let you be the judge. One of my staff sent me a link to a story about an InF vaccine they've developed."

"We knew that."

"But now everyone knows."

Antioch furrowed his brow. "Send me the link. Did you send it to Poseidon?"

"Sending it to both of you now, but it's all over the internet. Check your feeds. Sounds like we may not need Quito now."

When Antioch received the link, he clicked on it and was taken to the *Arizona Times Herald's* website.

Arizona Times Herald
SPECIAL EDITION
Sunday, July 18, 2021

Is This Horseshoe Close Enough?

Scientists have taken advantage of the resilient horseshoe crab to formulate a vaccine in just thirty-eight days that has shown the ability to not only stop the progression of the insomnia flu but reverse the devastating effects of the prion's influence on healthy proteins.

The bright blue blood of these helmet shaped Merostomata (an arthropod classification which means "legs attached to the mouth") coagulates when exposed to endotoxins. LAL appears to be the answer for our fifty-something-year-old citizens. When used as a medium into which monoclonal bodies are introduced, abnormal proteins such as the folded prion, with a lack of "prion food" or energy [see end note for details] fail to survive. Even previously folded proteins go through an "unfolding" process, restoring the affected victim to a normal healthy state.

There is one hiccup. Not only does the blood medium need to come from the species Tachypleus tridentatus, but from a specimen which contains a defective hemocyte.

Let's disentangle the above. This specific horseshoe crab was genetically predisposed to contain blood with twice the strength of other crabs and it took this to survive the unfolding process. The good news is, when fertilized, the eggs in this super-crab will hatch in nine days, when it usually takes two to four weeks. This horseshoe crab, named Tacky by one of the researchers after a penguin in her daughter's library, is living the good life. She is massaged daily, introduced to many beaus and is fed New Zealand cockle clams six times a day. Authorities are not disclosing her location at this time.

Questions remain, of course. What side effects will be seen, in both the short and long term? Has this been tested on enough patients to feel good about recovery? Will the vaccine fallout be worse than the disease? Speaking with an anonymous source familiar with the discovery, we have learned as long as the vaccine is used in an insomnia flu-infected individual, it should benefit the patient and very likely will cure them of the condition they were introduced to twenty years ago. However, they warn, extreme prejudice should be employed when not sure if the patient has contracted the insomnia flu. Further details will be provided later.

[2-DG, or 2-deoxy-D-glucose, is the molecule which makes up the "energy killer" found in horseshoe crab blood. 2-DG is differentiated from D-glucose by removing oxygen from the second carbon atom. Because it so closely mimics D-glucose, which gets free passage through the blood-brain barrier, the prion requires the metabolic process called glycolysis to survive. Specifically, D-glucose breaks down into three-carbon compounds, one of them being pyruvate anion ($CH3COCOO$) when energy is released. 2-DG, however, is incapable of going through glycolysis, so there is no energy available for the prions to sustain their march toward indiscriminately folding proteins]

When Will This Vaccine Be Available?

Officials with NIAID (National Institute of Allergy and Infectious Diseases) in partnership with the Department of Health and Human Services (HHS) are in communication with the Department of Defense (DoD) and the Centers for Disease Control (CDC) to coordinate supply, production, and distribution of the vaccines. The DoD contacted the Arizona Times Herald and asked us to pass on the following:

Questions relating to distribution of the new InF vaccination should be directed to one of the following resources:

InFVACC@DoD.org
844-VACCINE or by visiting
www.InFVACCINE.org

Antioch texted Poseidon and Falcon.

Poseidon. U know what to do.

Already in motion.

77

6:21 a.m.
Underground Lab Facility, Chandler Complex,
Department of Molecular and Cellular Biosciences,
University of Arizona

"We already have over six hundred emails to the DoD address,"
said Tom. "How the heck did you get that ported to us, Karla?"

Karla Mackin, like her sister Kira, never married. She was the
introverted sister. When most boys her age would spend hours each
day learning how to play the newest Nintendo 64 video game, Karla
was designing the next generation. Sony brought her on as a high
school sophomore to lead their game designer team, but she soon
grew bored, and, perhaps through a desire to join her sister and
father in public service, became an electronic warfare intelligence
specialist for a "signature reduction" force within the army.

Their professions took precedence over relationships, and
although Karla's high cheekbones and slender figure had brought
considerable attention, her true love was electronic intelligence,
or EI. She scoffed at artificial intelligence, saying, "There's nothing
artificial about what I do." If she had been truthful with herself,

it was her profession that unnerved those who would solicit her attention. Men, on the whole, would prefer to keep a few secrets.

"I've got friends at the DoD. Other than that, you're on a need-to-know basis, Tom." She meant this as a joke, but where she excelled in electronic espionage, she suffered in her delivery of humor.

Tom rotated uneasily to the computer and pulled up the web site visit data. "With the A.P. picking up the story, our site can't take much more, guys. We knew to be prepared, but I see a crash coming—"

"Not important," Jacob cut him off. "We got the phone call, and that's all that matters."

They had let all calls go to a voice mail greeting which said, "Due to overwhelming interest in the new insomnia flu vaccine, we are unable to take your call at this time, but your message will be received and reviewed, and if it warrants a return call, we will get back with you as soon as possible. You may also visit the FAQ section on www.InFVACCINE.org. Thank you."

The voice mail they waited for did not take long to come in.

"This is the Phoenix police department. We have reason to believe that the horseshoe crab known as Tacky is being held in the Phoenix/Tucson corridor, and we would like to help. We think when the location is eventually revealed to the public, you will see rioting and forceful entries. Please allow us to protect you. Call the number you see on the caller I.D. and please hurry."

When Karla called the police number back, she used a phone that would be traced to the lab and told the woman who answered the offer of protection was appreciated. She gave her the correct address, including the fact they would be in the underground lab.

On the third floor of the Civil Engineering building a few blocks away from the lab, Jacob gathered Marie, Kira, Sawyer, Luca, Kyle and Tom, but all eyes were on Karla now.

As they sat around a plexiglass table, she revisited the instructions for everyone and rechecked the readiness of the equipment. They passed the time for the next hour going over contingencies with some detours into Luca's past, Kyle's injured knee, and Marie's ability to metabolize alcohol so quickly.

"Here they come," Karla said. She had brought four prototype miniature stealth drones code-named Gawker which the Air Force beta tested recently. She had been asked to do some testing for them and she happily agreed. They were currently deployed over the four corners of the campus. The group watched the one hundred and fifty-inch 8K LED monitor on the wall as Karla scrolled through various shots from the drones as well as from cameras she had installed on building cornices thirty feet above street level. These cameras were made to resemble pigeons, down to the last detail. They would move their head from side to side, allowing the camera to scan a larger area, and every few minutes, they would release a thimble-sized white mass which would fall to the concrete below.

Karla now had twelve camera views on the large monitor. One from each drone and eight others. They were able to count fourteen squad cars and two unmarked black sedans arriving together. Once the contingency arrived, they split up and spread out around the campus. One of the black sedans parked near the campus entrance on Highland Avenue between the parking garage and the food pantry and idled. The other advanced, turning twice before arriving at the front entrance of the Chandler building which housed the underground lab.

They watched four men in uniforms step out. Two of them drew weapons and used the top of the opened car doors to stabilize their arms, which held Glock 19s and were aimed at the front door. The other two split. One walked toward the front door, and one appeared to head toward the back of the building. The man at the front entrance climbed the eight concrete steps in a measured but deliberate manner. Dark sunglasses kept the ten-thirty-sun from impeding his progress.

"You were right, Jacob," Luca said. "They suspect something."

Their eyes had been trained on the central actor, but Karla's experience kept her scanning all screens. "They've been ordered to drive toward the lab. See that car?" She pointed to a squad car on the screen advancing slowly. They nodded. "He's driving by this building right now."

"Glasses walked in," Sawyer said.

They watched all cars heading toward the lab. After another minute, Jacob said, "Here comes Montgomery."

The other unmarked sedan now maneuvered toward the lab. "How do you know that's Montgomery?" asked Kira.

"He wants to see this play out."

"He got a message from Glasses inside," said Karla. "He was just waiting for the safe call." She switched out four screens, which were the drones showing the periphery of the campus and substituted with four shots of the inside of the Chandler building. One showed the front door, one the stairwell leading to the basement, and two angles of the underground lab.

"But if they're expecting a trap—"

"Not a problem," said Jacob. "That's what we want." Activity on all screens rapidly picked up. Word surfaced there was something going down at the Chandler building. Although it was summer, seventeen buildings had classes in session and when students saw police cars from Phoenix drive past windows through which they frequently daydreamed, class was over.

Messages flew around campus, and little time passed before the streets around the Chandler building became a mixture of twenty-year-old postpubescent students and twenty-year-old postpubescent officers. From the motions and gestures, it was difficult to tell if the policemen were refusing to provide the students with information about the exercise or simply had no details to relate. The temperature topped one hundred degrees and was climbing, which mattered little to the assembly.

The IP cameras in the lab were disguised as alarm systems and had zoom capabilities to 36X. They were synched with the microphone Karla installed into a stapler on one of the lab desks. The officer who originally entered the building first was also the first through the lab door. He scanned the room, saw no sign of danger, then said into a mic clipped to his lapel, "You're not going to like this, sir."

Montgomery walked in a minute later, and his dispassionate expression quickly dissipated. "Bring in Major!" he shouted through gritted teeth. Another officer holding the leash of a white German Shepherd entered and released the beautiful animal. It quickly navigated all areas of the lab, stopped momentarily to sniff the drawers of a cabinet housing various reagents, then moved on until it completed its mission.

Montgomery pulled a cell phone out of his jacket pocket and punched a number. A speaker next to Karla three blocks away came to life.

"What have you got, Poseidon?"

"No one's here. No sign of any horseshoe crab either."

In the Civil Engineering Building blocks away, Kyle asked Karla, "You can record both sides of a cell phone conversation even when you're not on one of the phones?"

Karla smiled but said nothing. She was more interested in the other conversation.

"You trace the call?" a gravelly voice asked on the other end.

"Yes. It came from this location."

"That means they could be close. Have you searched the other buildings?"

"Not yet. We have a crowd now, but my men are mute."

"Good. Get a message out—"

"Wait. Hold on." He walked to the lab bench in the middle of the room and picked up a black stapler. He turned it over and grinned. "They've been listening in through a stapler, Anti . . . hanging up. I've got a message to send."

He brought the stapler close to his mouth. "Very clever, but very stupid. If you want to see Ms. Quito alive again, you'll give us the location of the crab. Oh, and for some extra credit, we have a miss Bailey Kasadam and two pretty boys. I'd hate to mess up any young faces."

Sawyer rose and paced frenetically. Sweat punched out of facial pores as he belted out a few unkind acts he would be exacting on Montgomery. "I know you're upset," said Jacob as he grabbed his arm and stopped his pacing. "But this is good news. You know they're alive now, and you know we have a plan."

Montgomery continued speaking into the stapler. "We'll give you one last chance to make this right. You've got the number to call. Eight hours. The younger boy gets the knife first." He laughed into the microphone, then threw the stapler against the brick wall as his laughter quickly turned to anger.

"There goes our audio," Karla said. They watched as Montgomery and Glasses stormed out of the building, got in their cars, and headed back to Phoenix. "Ain't it beautiful when a game plan works to perfection?"

"Everyone still up for this?" Jacob stood while Karla packed up her gear. The mood was somber with the knowledge they were dealing with people who were willing to perform barbaric acts on young children. No one wanted to respond enthusiastically with emotions in the balance, so they nodded and helped Karla load her Benz Sprinter which had the passenger seats removed for her trip back to Virginia.

With the van full and gear stowed, Karla handed an iPad to Jacob. "Password is Jared."

"Thanks. Can't tell you how much we appreciate your help."

"What help?" she asked as she stepped into the driver's seat. "I was never here." She shut the door and drove off. When she drove through Wilcox, she called the Phoenix police number she had called before.

"Phoenix Police Department," said the calm, breathy voice on the other end.

"I have a message for Chief Montgomery." Karla had activated a noise-cancelling feature on her phone which would not allow the person on the other end to hear car noise.

"He's listening."

"He can locate Tacky as well as some vaccine solution stored in a refrigerator in the back of an establishment called Baking with Betty on 27th Avenue. She shut the classes down a few months ago and I'm sure you'll be able to get in."

"And how do we know you're telling the truth? The stunt you pulled before cost us valuable time. People are dying every day."

"Tell us where you have the boys."

"You know we can't—"

"Exactly. Now that we know what you're willing to do to two innocent boys, we'd be fools to try anything again. The vaccine will be there with instructions on dosage. It needs to be kept at fifty-eight degrees, so if you intend to transport it, you'll need to prepare for that."

There was a pause. Karla assumed the messenger was communicating with Montgomery. After a minute, she returned. "Is this the only vaccine ready for use?"

"Yes, it is, and we hope you'll do the right thing and work with Tacky. She will need to be given a sandy beach to lay her eggs and male horseshoe crabs from the *Tachypleus tridentatus* family—at least thirty—will be needed to fertilize the millions of eggs she will lay." Karla waited for a response.

"I'm still here."

"You'll need a crab phlebotomist to drain her blood, but not enough to kill her. Then you'll need DNA samples from the eggs which will hatch in about ten days. You need to separate those that have the Hox-A and Hox-C on the 14th chromosome." Again, she waited.

"Anything else?"

It was obvious to Karla what they would be doing to Tacky . . . and Karla did not care because Tacky would be hundreds of miles away.

78

Montgomery removed the ear buds and dropped them into his pocket. He sat alone in the back seat as two officers escorted him back to the station. He picked up his cell phone and sent a text.

Having pancakes at 3:15.
Baking with Betty on 27th.

How many pancakes?

Only 3.

What if we're not hungry?

May be last chance for pancakes.

Will park on street and wait for you.

I'm in too. Do I bring 4 stooges?

Good idea.

Sandam put his phone in his pocket and walked down a dark narrow hall, which ended in a locked metal door. He peered through a peephole, which had been installed on the outside, and when satisfied with what he saw, unlocked the door, and went in. Bailey was propped up on pillows, legs out and crossed on the bed. She glared at the intruder when he entered.

"Gonna let us go home now?" she asked, arms folded in defiance.

Sandam grinned. "We're going on a field trip, but the destination is not your home. However, if we discover what we need, you have my word . . . you can go home."

"I suppose it's futile to ask what the hell you're talking about."

He ignored this, then turned to the two young boys who were busy playing Minecraft. "Boys, we're going for a ride."

Derrall paused the game. "Are you taking us to see our daddy?"

When Sandam did not immediately answer, Bailey pressed. "Well?"

"Come on, boys. It's a surprise."

Derrall still had his game paused but made no effort to move. "Are we playing the game where you tie up Aunt Bailey again?"

Sandam smiled. "I'll be back in five. I'll need you all to be ready to go." He eyed Bailey, gave her a no-nonsense glare, then walked out the door and locked it, turned, and strode down the long hallway. He extracted a hickory jumpsuit from a hall cabinet, walked outside through a pocket door, across a wooden bridge which spanned a kidney-shaped pool, and entered a room through glass doors.

It was sparsely furnished and resembled a large den which had been stripped of any personality in preparation for sale. There was no art on the walls, no tables, chairs, or lamps. The low rumble of central air was absent which created a dank, warm, and stifling environment. In the lone piece of furniture, a carrot-colored futon, sat Jilian Quito. She was now bald, the black stubble which remained all that was left of a beautiful eighteen inches of shiny onyx hair. An Ace bandage encircled her head and held a large patch of gauze that covered her wound. It was the only piece of fabric on her body.

When Sandam entered, she folded her hands in her lap to protect what little privacy she could. He tossed the jumpsuit next to her. "Get dressed," he demanded. When she failed to react, he warned, "Suit yourself. We're going for a ride, and if you want—"

As he leaned to pick up the clothing, Jilian snatched it, stood, and turned away from him as she slipped into the suit. "You know the drill," he said. She put her hands behind her back, and he quickly bound her wrists with duct tape. "Let's go." He held her arm as they left the room and walked down a stone path, which led to a private drive under a latticed portico. He opened the back door of a silver Lexus SUV and guided her in. He locked the car, then headed back to get the other three. He bound Bailey's hands using the same roll of duct tape and motioned them out the door. He used the remote to unlock the door and when he opened the back door to let Bailey in, she yelled, "Now!"

The two boys took off down the drive and headed toward the street as Jilian awkwardly jumped from the back seat onto the driveway. Sandam calmly withdrew a Ruger GP100 and aimed it at Jilian, who was attempting to rise with bound hands. "Bailey, I'm going to ask you this one time. Get the boys back here, or Ms. Quito here gets a bullet where she least wants one."

Bailey froze, not knowing what to do.

"Don't do it," Jilian pleaded.

Bailey waited another second, then shouted, "Derrall! Weldon! Come back! It's all right!" They had disappeared and she was not sure they could hear her. "Derrall! Weldon!" A few seconds later, they appeared and slowly walked back toward them. "Good boys! Hurry, now, we need to leave!" Bailey prayed she had made the right decision.

79

Ten miles away, the black sedan turned on to 27th and Montgomery said, "You can just drop me off, boys."

The driver investigated the rearview mirror, knowing he should not question his chief, then made the most prudent decision. "Yes, sir."

"Right here will be good." They were two blocks from the bakery, but the driver pulled to the curb and Montgomery got out. After he closed the door, he poked his head back through the open window. "You dropped me off at my house." They both nodded.

As he started up the street, he could see Governor Adair's 1966 Jaguar XJ13, which looked out of place in this zip code. When he reached it, he rapped on the passenger's window and Adair jumped.

"Hellfire, Monty!" he said as Montgomery opened the door and sat.

"Shouldn't bring this jag around here. Might lose some hubcaps."

Adair had the AC set to max, but sweat drops formed on his forehead. "No sign of Sandam yet. This almost over? My insomnia's picking up lately. This vaccine better be legit."

"They got an EUA. That's Emergency Use Authorization from HHS so it moved to a fast track. I was told it was very close to another one they were working on, so just a little tweaking got it done. I'm just as anxious as you, Governor. They also know we'll likely inject their women and maybe even the boys before we try it on ourselves, so I'm feeling good about it."

"Where's Sandam?"

On cue, the silver SUV pulled in behind the jaguar. They both got out, and Adair quickly used the remote to lock and arm his car.

Sandam stepped out of the Lexus and motioned Montgomery to go to the other side. Bailey stared through the window at the police chief, eyes ablaze. "Jeez, you had to gag her?"

Sandam opened the door on the other side to let Jilian out. "Couldn't get her to shut up. No choice." Jilian stepped out and he grabbed her arm. "Let's go, boys."

"Can't they stay in the car?" Jilian pleaded.

"Too hot out here. That would be very irresponsible of us, right, chief?"

Montgomery ignored him as he grabbed Bailey's arm and walked across the street to a storefront, which included four businesses. Baking with Betty was sandwiched between a nail spa and a shopping center church called Retro Jesus.

Montgomery's dark suit and the governor's sombrero, along with a sun umbrella be brought, drew modest attention from passersby. The chief removed Bailey's gag and placed a gun in the small of her back to ensure she made no scene. Both women had escorts to hide the fact their hands were bound. To anyone glancing their way, they appeared to be showing up for a cooking class with Betty. Derrall asked Adair why he was using an umbrella when it wasn't raining. The governor ignored the question like a seasoned politician.

Montgomery used his Sparrow's lock pick set and had the door open in seconds. "Ladies first." He and Sandam stood on either side of the door, both with guns raised. Adair stood twenty feet away under the nail spa awning and wiped sweat with his monogrammed handkerchief. The boys followed the women, Sandam flipped the light switch, and they began the search for a refrigerator. Seeing none, Sandam opened a door behind a Formica counter, which had seen considerable business over the years, but which now was topped with several layers of dust and turned on the light.

There was a large square table in the middle with a sink, and an antique pine top with shelving underneath. There were six refrigerators and two freezers lining the walls. Three of the refrigerators had glass doors and three metallic. Montgomery kept a gun trained on the women while Sandam opened each one. When the third door opened, he smiled. On one shelf sat a chrome box with a red piece of tape holding down the lid. On the front was a sticker from Health and Human Services and another from the FDA.

The shelf below held a rectangular glass aquarium with no water, but in which sat a horseshoe crab. A piece of masking tape with the name *Tacky* was attached to the front of the glass.

To the left of the aquarium was a paper sack. Before he opened it, he turned toward Montgomery and said, "You can remove their restraints, but lock the door first." He locked the door and cut away the tape on their wrists with a hunting knife he pulled out of nowhere. The ladies rubbed their wrists to return some missing circulation. Sandam removed the sack from the shelf and handed it to Bailey. "Open it."

She took it, unfolded the top and inspected the interior. "No snake."

Sandam grabbed it from her and pulled out a lined piece of paper that had been torn off a pad. He read it aloud for Montgomery and Adair.

"You will find a set of twelve disposable syringes in the bag. Withdraw one cc of the vaccine through the rubber vial top, ensuring the solution is clear and uncontaminated and inject into muscle. The deltoid is the preferred location. Expect a sore arm and potential nausea, chills, fever and fatigue over the initial twelve hours."

He pulled the box off the shelf and laid it on the table. Using Montgomery's knife, he slit the tape, then slid the box across the table. "Would you do us the honor?" he asked Jilian.

She opened the flaps and sniffed. "No cyanide gas," then slid it back to Sandam.

He removed an opaque, gray container with a velcroed lid. He averted his gaze as he opened it, then returned and found twelve smaller, opaque, gray containers with red, circular rubber inserts in the top of each one. He pulled one out and set it on the table, removed a disposable syringe from the bag, removed the cap and withdrew clear liquid to the two-cc mark.

"This won't hurt at all," he said as he walked toward Bailey.

"What the hell is that?" betraying the confident behavior she had shown to this point. As she backed away, Montgomery grabbed Weldon and placed the barrel of his gun against his temple.

"No!" she screamed. "All right! Shoot me up with whatever you want!"

"That's better," Sandam said corrosively.

Bailey shut her eyes and allowed him to inject the vaccine into her arm. "What now, Mr.—"

"Sandam," Jilian interjected. "That's Kevin Sandam."

"I don't know who that's supposed to be, but I know that's our sorry-ass governor in the corner over there trying to not be recognized. So, what happens now, dipstick? Do I start growing horns and rotatin' my head?"

"I'm ready for you to put her gag back in," said Adair quickly.

"She's served her purpose, Antioch," said Montgomery. "Why don't you shut her up for good?"

"Not in front of the kids," Adair interjected.

"We need to wait it out a little longer," said Sandam. "Until we know the vaccine is safe." He turned toward Bailey. "Count backwards from a hundred." When she just stared at him, he said, "Don't make me—"

"One hundred, ninety-nine, ninety-eight, ninety-seven, ninety-six, ninety-five, ninety-four, ninety-three, ninety—"

"That's good enough. Now bend over and touch your toes." When she did this with ease, he said, "Guys. I say we get this over with and get out of here. The crab's cute, but he needs to meet our woodchipper."

"I'll take care of that," said Montgomery.

Sandam took three more containers out, along with three more syringes and prepared each one.

"I'll go first," said Adair. "I can't get rid of this insomnia soon enough."

"Is that what this is all about?" asked Jilian. "The vaccine?"

Ignoring her, he walked over to the table and pulled up his sleeve. Sandam injected the vaccine, then did the same with Montgomery, who then gave Sandam his injection.

"What do we do with them now?" asked Adair.

"Can't do anything here," said Sandam. "Too many eyes were on us when we came in. I suggest we get things cleaned up, make sure our finger . . . prints . . . are . . . uh." He leaned against the table to steady himself. He lifted his head with difficulty and saw Montgomery and Adair were doing the same. He fell to his knees, thinking they had been tricked, but then saw Jilian collapse as well, just before he fell to the floor, closed his eyes, and went to sleep.

Within a few minutes, Jacob, Sawyer, Tom and Luca walked in the room wearing tactical gas masks. It took them ten minutes to get the dead weight of Jilian, Bailey and the boys into the van without arousing suspicion. When this was accomplished, Marie used Tom's mask and went into the back room to write a note. She impaled it over the ferrule of Adair's umbrella while Kira used Sawyer's mask to retrieve the rest of the vaccines and Tacky's cousin. "Night boys!" she said as she flipped off the light and met the others in the van.

"Wait!" Sawyer said. "I forgot something." He replaced his mask, hurried back inside, and walked over to the sedated Sandam. "This is from my boys." Using his steel-toed boot, he kicked him in the mouth, fracturing all four of his upper incisors. He then walked over to Montgomery and with considerable force, brought his heel down on an exposed right hand, breaking four fingers in several places. Finally, he found the governor and kicked him in the groin, then walked back to the van.

As they sped away, Kyle inspected the arms of the four sleeping passengers. "Apparently, Bailey is the only one they injected."

"Damn," said her brother. "She was probably mouthing off."

"It's all right, Sawyer," said Luca. "She'll be fine." He pulled a vial out of a bag next to him and filled a syringe with the contents. Jacob pulled the Ford E-Transit van over to the shoulder and flipped on the emergency flashers. When it came to a stop, Luca moved to the seat Bailey was laying on and injected her arm with the solution. Like the others, she would be out for a while . . . and wouldn't remember anything from this evening. No one asked Sawyer what he forgot.

80

At 2:14 a.m., Montgomery's eyes opened like apathetic garage doors. At first, he could not move, and he thought it was another bout of sleep paralysis he had experienced since his twenties. Then he felt severe pain in his right hand but could not move yet. When he regained some muscle tone, he tried to flex his hand and screamed in agony. When he was able to sit, he also realized the right side of his head must have been injured. He felt a bump above his ear with his left hand and winced. He felt no moisture in his hair to indicate bleeding, but it was too dark to see.

His eyes began to adjust, but with no windows to usher in the leftovers from streetlamps, he slowly crawled on one hand and both knees to explore the surroundings. He had no idea where he was and no memory of how he got here. A thin light escaped from one of the refrigerators and he crawled toward it. When he reached it, he opened the door, which cast light into the dark room.

Across the room, he saw someone moving, struggling as he had. "Kevin, is that you? Sandam?"

Now that there was light to guide him, Montgomery stood shakily, held on to the refrigerator door, then worked his way toward the distressed man. He assured himself that indeed this was Kevin Sandam, then turned on the light switch. Only then did he hear snoring on the other side of the baker's table. Sandam was now sitting up. "What the hell?"

"I was gonna ask you the same question, Kevin. Oh my god. You've got some broken teeth!"

Sandam reached up and felt where his teeth should have been. When he spoke, his words were garbled. "What a uck ha-enned"?

"Hey, my hand's in bad shape, and my head has a knot. Could we have collapsed here? Our falls created the injuries? Do you remember anything?" Sandam shook his head in disbelief, holding his mouth and finally realizing the throbbing pain that emanated from four exposed nerves.

Montgomery walked over to the snorer and realized it was Governor Adair, then hissed through gritted teeth. "Potter."

"Can't be," said Sandam. "He's dead."

"Have you seen the body? Have we seen *any* of the bodies from the fire?"

"I don't guess you know how we got here?"

"I'm gonna get some answers," Montgomery seethed. "We'd better wake up lard-ass."

Sandam was still leaning on the table for support. Montgomery walked over to a sink, found a water pitcher in the cabinet, and filled it with water. When he returned, he emptied the contents on Adair's face and torso. The snoring stopped, but he made no effort to move.

"Is he breathing, Monty?"

"Just barely. Sleeping without that CPAP machine ain't good for his beauty sleep."

Sandam chuckled with little enthusiasm. Standing with a little more confidence, he said, "I don't know where we are or how we got here, but we need to lea. Might just lea him here. I'm not carrying him."

"He might remember something, Kevin. We can't—"

They heard Adair groan and turn onto his side.

Sandam reacted. "Gonah! Wake up! You missed Christmas!"

Adair tried raising an arm but failed. In unison, they walked over to help him up. They got him to a sitting position in time to see him trying to lift his eyelids. Failing this, he said, "Where am I and why am I all wet?"

"You peed yourself, guvnah," said Montgomery.

"Not funny." Then he grabbed his genitals, which were aching.

"Too bad you didn't ha your umbrella up. It must ha rained on you." Sandam glanced over at the unfolded rain shade parked against the wall and saw a piece of paper attached to it. He pulled it off the point and began reading to himself, then decided to read out loud with altered diction necessitated by some missing teeth. He particularly struggled with his f's and v's.

"You hae all been injected with the accine or the insomnia lu. Congratulations. Check your arms to erify this."

Adair was aware enough now to join the others in feeling of their arms. They eyed each other and nodded.

"We hae let enou accine or you to test—"

"Give that to me, Sandam. I can barely understand you." Montgomery grabbed it with his left hand and continued.

"We have left enough vaccine for you to test if you so choose. If you are looking for Tacky, he is safe. An exposé has been written which details the machinations of the Klavian Triumvirate. This is poised to be sent to all news outlets around the U.S., but you can prevent this by standing down. If we see any evidence that you are working to prevent us from erasing the genocide you have put in motion, the message goes out. YSA."

81

Back at Kyle's lake house, day was breaking. Red-throated loons Dr. Hunter had shipped from Canada two years before, yodeled from the far side of the lake, where the water was more comfortable, and shade from a southern magnolia protected them from the morning sun. Kyle had placed twelve aerators, six Aquaforce pumps, and three waterfalls to keep the water temperature down, but the northern birds still complained.

Sawyer had been out for a swim and trudged back up the hill toward the house, shaking the water from some blond locks. The young boys awoke from their sedation first, at around 4:00 a.m., but went back to sleep. Bailey and Jilian had soon followed but remembered no events since their time in the Civil Engineering Building in Tucson. Kyle and Jacob filled in the blanks the best they could.

"You mentioned the gas," said Bailey, "but I feel like I'm missing some details."

Luca offered to explain. "One of our projects, if you want to call it that, when Enzo and I were playing around as grad students, was to perfect flunitrazepam."

"Fluni what?"

"Rohypnol. The date rape drug."

"No, you didn't," Jilian piped in.

"Don't worry. It wasn't about the girls. We were geeks, remember?" He hoped for some dissentient affirmations here which never came. "Anyway, it had never been turned into a gas form, but we used the cow as a model, or actually, a vehicle. It eats biomass such as grass or hay and uses its intestines to produce biogas. We had a lot of fun feeding Rohypnol—putting it in their hay—to cows and watching them fall asleep. We then, and don't ask me how we did this, but we collected the gas, separated out the methane and were left with pure flunitrazepam gas. We then realized when compressed, the gas liquefied."

"You really are a geek," said Bailey.

"I take that as a compliment," Luca said, smiling.

"And what was that about the CPAP?" Jilian asked.

Marie jumped in. "With CPAP machines, or PAP machines to be more generic, there's usually a humidifier filled with distilled water to moisten the air before it enters the nose."

"My mother had one of those," said Sawyer. "She never even took a nap without it."

"It's a lifesaver for many," Marie said. "Anyway, a few million of them were recalled, and we had patients bringing them in to us, thinking we could replace them. Of course, we couldn't, but we found a good use for one of them."

Luca broke in. "We put the Rohypnol in a cylinder and compressed it, then inserted it into the PAP machine in place of the humidifier. We used a fifty-foot neoprene gas hose from Jacob's grill setup and used good old duct tape to attach it to the CPAP hose. Then we fed it through—"

"We?" Sawyer interjected.

"All right, *Sawyer* climbed in the attic and ran the hose through the ductwork just shy of the vent in the baking room—"

"By the way," Sawyer interrupted. "Those air ducts? They're nothing like you see in the movies. There's no perfectly squared off clean metal to elbow through."

"All the same, thanks for doing that, Sawyer. This fat boy would have never negotiated that. So as soon as we knew everyone was in the room—Kyle was our spotter across the street in the Scuba Toys dive shop—he had to wear a mask and snorkel for like an hour. Anyway, as soon as he messaged Marie, she turned on the PAP machine."

"But you said they gave each other the vaccines," Kira said. How did you time it?"

"We were lucky," said Marie. "Flunitrazepam gas, just like the original date rape drug, has no taste, and is odorless, so we knew it really didn't matter when it took effect, but even if they hadn't injected each other with the vaccine, we could have done it for them."

"So," Jilian started. "Since we can't remember any of this, and I understand that's what Rohypnol does, but does that mean they don't remember anything either? I mean Montgomery, Sandam and Adair."

"That's correct," said Sawyer. "And thankfully, Marie didn't sign her name to that note."

Jacob walked out the back door and joined them on the patio, carrying Tom's open laptop. "The press release we wrote already has 12,089 views."

"What does it say?" asked Bailey.

He laid the computer in front of her so she could read it.

VIADERA InF-21 VACCINE AUTHORIZED FOR USE IN AFFECTED ADULTS AGED 50-59

August 3, 2021, Phoenix—The Centers for Disease Control and Prevention (CDC) reviewed the recommendations of the Advisory Committee on Immunization Practices (ACIP) and today endorsed the use of Viadera InF-21 Vaccine for adults aged 50-59 and others confirmed to have contracted the insomnia flu.

The CDC approval follows Monday's Emergency Use Authorization (EUA) by the U.S. Food and Drug Administration. In a risky and potentially controversial move which dramatically shortened the timeline, the CDC removed safety hurdles which had been in place since the Cutter incident in 1954 when the Division of Biologic Standards was formed to oversee vaccine safety. Some are saying this "shadow-docket" circumvention of procedural safeguards is ethically irresponsible, but with over 42 million adults at risk, many of whom are end-stage victims, and with the help of the lowly horseshoe crab who made it possible to reverse the degradation or folding of healthy proteins, the vaccine was approved with the following contraindications and precautions.

– - - the following has been truncated for space purposes - - –

- The InF vaccine must be administered only to those infected with the InF virus. In adults without the InF prions present, live, attenuated vaccine will lead to another protein misfolding disorder— immunoglobulin light chain amyloidosis. Life expectancy is less than one year with this gatecrashing disease, so a definitive diagnosis is paramount.
- Women known to be pregnant should not receive live, attenuated vaccines.
- Severe combined immunodeficiency disease (SCID).
- Intussusception.

- See www.InFVaccine.org/contraindications for expanded details.

DISTRIBUTION

To illustrate why the endorsed vaccine was expedited by the CDC and FDA, there are currently 14,000 hatchlings from the horseshoe crab known as Tacky, who has both Hox-A and Hox-C found on her 14th chromosome. Half of these are female. Can these 7,000 females lay eggs to help us out? Yes, but that will not happen until they mature—in ten years. Therefore, it is only Tacky's offspring whose blood can be used as the medium for the InF vaccine. But do we really have 14,000 horseshoe children of Tacky who can participate in the bloodletting? Hardly. The unusual 14th chromosome is X-linked recessive. Only 25% of the 14,000 will contain the genetic code necessary, so there are but 3500 in the pipeline. A piece of good news amongst the doom? Tacky can lay another 40,000 eggs next week. In total, she will give us 144,000 eggs, 60,000 of which will be successfully fertilized, giving us 15,000 horseshoe crabs to save over 40 million lives. In ten years, when these hatchlings are mature enough to mate, the epidemic will have ended. This is why extreme care is being taken to protect the eggs from predators and temperature fluctuations. Maximizing the number of Tacky's kids whose blood we can use is the number one focus.

Finally, during the early days of the insomnia flu, as we have seen in these times when fact and fiction have been unconscionably conflated, we list below the side effects which, though promulgated online as well as in our own paper as truth, we can unequivocally state are untrue.

- Imagined (or actual) levitation
- Weight loss in toes
- Loss of frontal hair (torso and pubic area)
- Humming Beatles songs at inappropriate times

Over the next few months, the insomnia flu vaccine made possible by the unlikeliest of characters, Tacky the horseshoe crab, brought debilitated quinquagenarians the healing power of sleep, erasing a decades-long effort to stem a growing population by mercilessly killing Americans in their most productive and contented years. Jacob Potter, after receiving a vaccine himself, moved the *Arizona Times Herald* into a newly built high rise which overlooked Camelback Mountain, but no one would write about Jacob's part in the eradication of the insomnia flu. He would not allow it.

Much speculation was offered as to the mysterious ailments of three prominent citizens. By Thanksgiving, the governor, the police chief, and a former aide to the governor were all hospitalized and on respirators. "They won't make it to see 2022," said a hospitalist who chose to remain anonymous.

They met again at Dr. Hunter's lake house and sat on the back porch enjoying the sixty-degree weather on an early December morning. Kyle had removed all the clocks in the house the day before in deference to Jacob. Jilian's facial lacerations and bruises were almost healed. Sawyer brought his redheaded attractive girlfriend, Reagan to join Jacob, Kyle, Marie, Luca, Jilian, and Kira for a last meeting before Luca moved back home to the Veneto area.

"Thanks for letting us use your home again, Kyle," Jacob started.

"Of course. Any time."

"I'll keep this short—just a few items on the agenda. Oh, and welcome, Reagan. Much of what we discuss won't make much sense—"

"Oh, I think it will," interrupted Sawyer. "I've filled her in pretty well."

"It sounds like the summer of twenty-one was pretty exciting for this group," Reagan said. "Maybe someday I can tell you about an eventful summer I had in Tulum."

Sawyer was proud of Reagan's humility. They had met on a plane trip back from Cancun, but before he contacted her later, he searched for her online. She had been profiled originally in a Tulum, Mexico editorial, and the story got picked up by numerous publications. A story emerged of her efforts at destroying a mafia kingpin in retaliation for her brother's death. He laughed to himself with her description of an "eventful" summer.

"Sounds interesting," Jacob said. "So first, Kyle, I'm anxious to hear what you figured out about Kevin Sandam."

"Ah yes. Ever since I remembered him changing his name over twenty years ago—he was a patient in my Dad's practice." He scanned the listeners who nodded. "For those who don't know, his name was Alex Bergfield until 1996 when for some unexplained reason he changed it to Kevin Sandam. I couldn't locate any other Sandams so I tried rearranging some letters and found you can rearrange Kevin Sandam to make 'Save Mankind.'"

"He picked a barbaric and twisted method for doing so," Marie said.

They all shook their heads in disbelief. "Luca," Jacob said. "You told us a little about how you were going to use the hair-loss experiments with the monkeys but fill in the details for us."

"Right. So, I pretended to be Governor Adair's assistant and began calling the top cognac distilleries asking for the next shipment date for the governor so we could make sure he would be in town to receive it. The first three, when they said they showed no orders from any Mr. Adair, I just said 'I'm terribly sorry. I'm embarrassed to say he told me to check, and I didn't ask which distillery.' I finally called Bache Gabrielsen and found his next shipment would be in two weeks. I then contacted a friend in Bordeaux. It's not too far from Cognac, France, and he owed me a favor, but when I told him what I was doing and why, he happily agreed to help."

"You're making me thirsty," said Jacob.

"My friend agreed to apply for a job at Bache Gabrielsen as a driver after their regular driver fell asleep at the wheel and crashed into a tree."

Sawyer asked, "How did you—"

"Doesn't matter. Things happen for mysterious reasons. I'll leave it at that." He grinned widely. "I shipped some of the Bongyloides stercoralis critters to—let's call him Pierre, along with some syringes which could penetrate the cork. He was able to locate the shipment going to Adair and injected the little guys into each bottle."

"This was how," Jacob offered, "we were able to convince the butchers they had the virus. They started losing hair about the time we published anecdotal reports of hair loss with the insomnia flu."

"I have a picture in my mind now that I can't erase," Reagan remarked. This brought smiles to the group.

"We knew the letter we sent telling them they had smelled the prion-saturated plant was not enough to convince them." Luca said. "In fact, we're not even sure the letter got to them."

"I almost forgot!" Jacob held up his index finger. "I had a difficult time reconciling how a group of men could rationally make the decision to kill millions of people using population control as the backdrop for their sins. Turns out they had a much bigger reason. Anyone ever heard of 60orBust.com?"

"Didn't the FBI start an investigation into that site recently?" asked Kyle.

"Yes, but what we found out yesterday is where the money was being funneled. Any guesses?"

"Wow. Didn't I read something like a hundred million in an offshore account?" Kyle's dad had called him from Belize with the news, joking that he could make a withdrawal in the International Bank there where the Triumverate was hiding their spoils.

"Excuse me," said Luca, "but what's this all about?"

Kyle held out his hand to Jacob, turning the floor over to the manager of the *Arizona Times Herald*.

"The site's been shut down by the FBI already so don't bother trying to find it, but it was a clever way to make money off people who would be dying in their fifties. People in their forties who had been sent a plant in their thirties were contacted five years ago. If you were forty-eight, for example, you could bet any amount you want, and if you made it to your sixtieth birthday, you would be sent 100 times your wager. So, if you were a healthy forty-five-year-old and your parents were alive in their seventies, you'd feel pretty good about investing ten thousand, for example, knowing you would then make one million when you hit sixty."

"Wait," Marie said. "How did they get them to invest before they were . . . like fifty-eight?"

"Great question. You had an account number keyed to your social. The countdown started at age forty-five, when you would make the one hundred x. Each year after that, your multiple would drop by twenty percent. If you waited until your forty-sixth birthday, you would only make eighty x. It was an ingenious way to get people betting on themselves early."

"Will they be able to get their money back?" asked Jilian.

Kyle shook his head. "If they do, it will be a while. Ultimately, the funds could be allocated to the families of those who have already died from InF. Could be years before it's all sorted out."

The group seemed stunned at the news, not knowing how to respond. They reflected silently on those who were slain so young and on those with an inexistent moral compass.

"One more question," Jacob said. "Or should I say statement. Not much has been made of the reason seventy-two percent of InF victims were female. Most assumed it was because more women were likely to keep plants, but Marie discovered something else we might want to use to tie this up with a bow. You have the floor."

"Yes, it didn't make sense to me. My boyfriend, Florian, loves plants more than I do, so I did some digging and found a study out of Brazil in 2014 which showed women have fifty percent more neurons in their olfactory bulbs, so they, for example, would enjoy the smell of a fragranced plant, leading them to take big sniffs."

"Is that why Wendy always complains—"

"Don't go there," said Kira.

Jacob smiled, then rose and pulled a bottle of champagne and a set of glasses out of the bag he had brought. "Finally," he said as he unwound the wrapper, "I have an announcement." He popped the cork and filled the glasses as he continued. "With the burning of the building which was home to the *Arizona Times Herald* for close to a century, I've made the decision to retire from the publishing business. I don't see this going on for another twenty years anyway, and I want to get ahead of that transition and not be caught in the eventual collapse. Sitting in the dark, observing the remains—the ashes of the building—I worried we had lost Jilian. It gave me a new perspective. I'm not sure what I'll do right now. Just going to take a sabbatical after the end of the year and see where it takes me. I'll let the *Arizona Times Herald* team know tomorrow but wanted my friends here to get first crack at telling me how stupid I am, so raise your glasses!"

They raised them high. "To a new beginning . . . and a year of excitement, recovery, and of making new friends. Salud!"

As the evening wound down and memories were shared, Jacob Potter said his farewells, then walked to his car. On his way, he keyed in "Change" by Taylor Swift for his gait song.

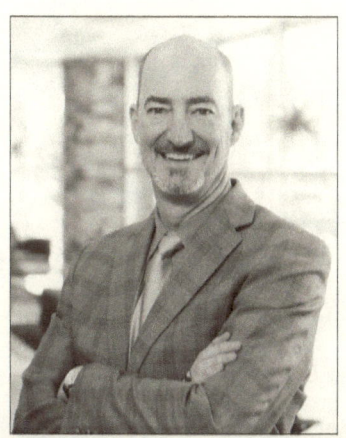

ABOUT THE AUTHOR

Dr. B Kent Smith has treated ten thousand sleep patients over the last twenty-seven years. He uses his experience, patient stories, and a healthy helping of imagination to weave this fictional story of sleep and the debilitating effect it can have for those deprived. His first novel is *The Unfortunate Gift*. Learn more about Dr. Smith on www.ksmithbooks.com or find him on Instagram or Facebook.

www.ingramcontent.com/pod-product-compliance
Lightning Source LLC
Chambersburg PA
CBHW032143190626
46814CB00005BA/1814